BEAT DIABETES

Dr. Peter Goh
Award-winning Laparoscopic and Metabolic Surgeon
Award-winning Author

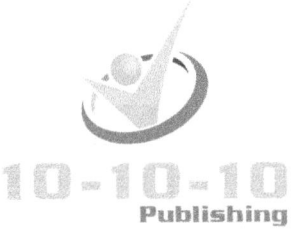

Beat Diabetes
Copyright © 2020 Dr. Peter Goh

ISBN: 978-1-67059-298-9

All rights reserved. No portion of this book may be reproduced mechanically, electronically, or by any other means, including photocopying, without permission of the publisher or author except in the case of brief quotations embodied in critical articles and reviews. It is illegal to copy this book, post it to a website, or distribute it by any other means without permission from the publisher or author.

Limits of Liability and Disclaimer of Warranty
The author and publisher shall not be liable for your misuse of the enclosed material. This book is strictly for informational and educational purposes only.

Warning – Disclaimer
The purpose of this book is to educate and inform. Although all information in this book is based on information from peer reviewed published scientific data the author and publisher do not guarantee that anyone following these techniques, suggestions, tips, ideas and strategies would have a successful outcome as medicine is still an inexact science and individual variation can occur. Individual patients will need to be managed by a bariatric/ metabolic surgeon to maximize the chance of success. The author and/or publisher shall have neither liability nor responsibility to anyone with respect to any loss or damage caused, or alleged to be caused, directly or indirectly by the information contained in this book.

Medical Disclaimer
The medical and or health information in this book is provided as an information resource only and is not to be used or relied on for any diagnostic or treatment purpose without the supervision of a bariatric/metabolic surgeon. This information is intended to be for patient education only and does not create any patient physician relationship and should not be used as a substitute for professional diagnosis and treatment.

Publisher
10-10-10 Publishing
Markham, ON   Canada

Printed in Canada and the United States of America

Table of Contents

Dedication	v
Foreword	vii
Preface	ix
Chapter 1: The Size of the Diabetes Problem	1
Chapter 2: What Can Diabetes Do to You?	7
Chapter 3: What Are the Types of Diabetes, and What Are Their Causes?	17
Chapter 4: Wish List for Those with Type 2 Diabetes	25
Chapter 5: Controlling Diabetes by Lifestyle Management	31
Chapter 6: Is Medicine the Solution?	45
Chapter 7: Insulin: The Curse of the Needles	51
Chapter 8: How Does Surgery Reverse Diabetes?	57
Chapter 9: What Procedures Can Reverse or Cure Diabetes?	67
Chapter 10: The Conquest of Fear	77
Chapter 11: The Surgery and Aftermath from the Patient's Point of View	87
Chapter 12: Pre-Diabetes – Don't Ignore It	95
Chapter 13: Why Obesity Must Be Reversed	
Chapter 14: Politics and Economics in the Diabetes World	103
Chapter 15: The Road to Reversing Diabetes – My Personal Journey	115
Chapter 16: Change the Game	135
About the Author	139
Acknowledgements	141

*This book is dedicated to Sonia Von Goh
Till we meet again.*

Foreword

Beat Diabetes by Dr. Peter Goh will change your life and make a difference to your health. It may even give you 10 or more extra years.

I met Dr. Goh two years ago in Singapore, and was immediately fascinated by his game-changing innovation of metabolic surgery. Diabetes, hypertension and other chronic diseases have for decades been considered incurable diseases which required life-long medication. This is no longer true.

Metabolic surgery has revolutionized the approach to chronic diseases. A simple one to two hour key-hole procedure can reverse Diabetes, often within days. This development will turn the medical world upside down.

Dr. Goh is the World pioneer for laparoscopic gastrectomy. He did the first operation in February 1992 and it was published in scientific journals and presented at the SAGES meeting in Washington DC in April 1992. This innovation was the building block upon which all gastric bypass operations were developed.

He has operated in more than 25 countries in 5 continents and is at present trying to bring the benefits of metabolic surgery to China and Russia.

He passionately preaches his message and I strongly urge you to read this book if you have Type 2 diabetes. There is a bright light at the end of the tunnel.

Raymond Aaron
New York Times Bestselling Author

Preface

Why do I need another book on diabetes?

Why, indeed? This subject has been written to death, and there are tons of material on the internet and social media. The problem is that there is so much clutter and fake news that the poor diabetic patient is totally confused by conflicting points of view. He is inundated with so much advice that it is impossible to distill all this information into a clear line of action that he can apply to his own situation.

So... let's cut through the fog and present the most important information, and give the patient, who is the most important person in the equation, just enough information to make some important choices.

In this book, everything stated is backed up by scientific studies and is published in mainstream, medical peer reviewed journals. Despite this, many people, especially those in the medical and pharmaceutical industry, will not agree with what are facts that are beyond dispute. Even if they agree, they are disinclined to bring attention to the true facts, because of vested interest.

The reasons they disagree are myriad, and I will try my best to wade through the priorities of all the interest groups involved.

In the end, the decision of what to do about your disease is yours, and yours alone. Whatever choice you make will result in consequences that you alone have to bear.

Beat Diabetes

There is no pill; there is no miracle cure and no magic bullet, but there is a near magical solution to all your problems. The question is, are you brave enough and decisive enough to grab it with both hands and reap the benefits today, before your disease slowly erodes your health and life away, as inexorably as climate change is degrading the world we live in.

In the end, I will point you to salvation.

A life without pills or injections is possible. You can, and you will, get back to normal, or almost, and turn back the tide of this chronic and potentially fatal disease. In the end, the news is good, and there is light at the end of the tunnel.

Before that, there is a short journey of enlightenment, and you must understand the adversaries you face.

OK. Please don't skip to the end of the book. There are many things you must understand before you get there. It is not a long journey, and the solution is far easier than you think.

Sit back and read, and let us take you on a little journey to put your life back in order, and make your life and health great again!

So, back to the question: Why do I need another book on diabetes? Answer: **The game has changed!**

Chapter 1

The Size of the Diabetes Problem

There are 500 million people in the world today with diabetes. This is almost as many people as the USA and Russia combined. The number is increasing rapidly, and many more are pre-diabetic, with a raised blood sugar level not yet necessitating medication. Then there are all the undiagnosed diabetics. These are people who don't even know they have the disease because they haven't checked their sugar levels. One study of global prevalence, published in 2013, surveying 130 countries, estimated a prevalence of 382 million, rising to 592 million by 2035.

Next to the common cold, this could be the most common condition we are facing. The number is rising; and by 2050, it would probably be double. Most countries have a prevalence rate of about 10%. In many countries, this is much more. According to the CDC, the prevalence of type 2 diabetes, in the USA in 2016, was 8.6%, or 21 million adults. For type 1 diabetes, it was 0.55%, or 1.3 million adults. That gives a ratio of about 93% having type 2, and 7% having type 1. The state with the highest rate of diabetes is West Virginia, at 15%, and it also has the highest rate of obesity (38.1%). The races that rank the highest are American Indians and Alaska natives, at 15.1%. Non-Hispanic whites have the lowest prevalence, at 7.4%. The cost of diabetes to the USA, in 2015, was $622.3 billion. This will increase by 53% in 2030. There are an estimated 8.1 million undiagnosed diabetics, which means that about one in three, or one in four, are undiagnosed.

Beat Diabetes

In many countries, this figure is much higher. China, for instance, had a prevalence of 11.9% of the adult population, in 2017, and the figure is rising so rapidly that it is posing a threat to their entire health system. By 2040, there will be 150 million diabetics in China. Four out of five adolescents in China are not getting enough exercise. In China, 109.6 million people have diabetes, and they have seen a sharp increase in the last 3 decades.

One of the highest prevalence of type 2 diabetes is seen in Malaysia, where 20.8% of adults above the age of 30 have the disease, which works out to 2.8 million people. The reasons are probably a high sugar and high carbohydrate diet based on rice, lack of exercise, and an inadequately funded health care system. A runaway obesity problem is another cause.

India is going to be the most populous country in the world. It will overtake China in 2020. There were already 73 million cases of diabetes recorded in India, in 2017. This is despite many Indians being vegetarian. Here again, obesity and lack of exercise are big factors, along with a largely rice and bread-based diet. The cultural factors also play a part. In India, obesity is considered a sign of prosperity. The poor people are largely thin, and the rich people are more likely to be fat, which is opposite of the North American situation, where the rich are health conscious and slim, and the lower economic group survives on fast food, have little opportunity to exercise, and are hence more likely to be obese. The prevalence of diabetes in India is 8.8%. The average age of onset is 42.5 years. One million Indians die from diabetes every year, and the total number of cases is 72 million!

Japan is a very interesting example of genes playing a major role. The Japanese, on the whole, are not fat; yet they have a relatively high rate of diabetes, at 12.1% (16.3% in men, and 9.3% in women). It is a relatively large population that is health conscious with a very healthy diet. The diet consists mainly of rice, fish, and vegetables, and the cooking style uses little fat or oil. Of course, American fast food has made inroads in their culinary culture.

In Europe, there are 60 million diabetics in the European region (10.3% of men, and 9.6% of women, have diabetes). Prevalence is increasing due to obesity, unhealthy diet, and physical inactivity. The lowest prevalence is in the Baltic states (Lithuania and Estonia) and Ireland, with about 4%, followed by Sweden and Luxembourg, at around 5%. One wonders what these countries are doing right. Is it genes or the right diet? Germany has the biggest population in Western Europe, with over 80 million people, and it has 7.5 million diabetics, which is average.

The prevalence rate in Russia is also relatively low, at 7.9%. There are 106 million Russian adults and about 8.5 million diabetics. When we look at the age group above 40, the rate rises to 11.7%, which is comparable to China and the USA.

Indonesia, with a population of 270 million, has about 16 million diabetics, but it is estimated that half of diabetics in Indonesia remain undiagnosed, especially young people, because of the lack of screening. I think the problem is about to explode there as well. Indonesia has a young population, with 42% of the population under 25, and 84% under 55, so we are just seeing the beginning of the problem. One in every 5 diabetics are now being diagnosed before the age of 40.

In South and Central America, the prevalence ranges from 8 to 11.3% of the adult population. Once again, there are a lot of undiagnosed cases (39%), so actual prevalence is probably double. Brazil (8.7%) has the most diabetics in this region, with about 12.5 million cases. Puerto Rico has the highest incidence, at 15.9%. Also high are Cuba (10.8%), Nicaragua (9.5%), Costa Rica (9.5%), and Chile (9.2%).

Peru and Ecuador are the lowest, with 5.2%, followed by Honduras (5.6%) and Argentina (5.8%). Actually, this region seems to show a huge variation between individual countries.

These countries have the lowest rates of diabetes in the world, and they are worthy of study: Azerbaijan (2.6%), Georgia (2.6%), Moldovia (2.5%), Gambia 2.0%), and Mali (1.6%)—and the prize goes to Benin, with 1.5%. So the area between the Black and Caspian Seas seems to have special features, and so does a smattering of West African countries.

On the other end of the scale are the top 8, which are Saudi Arabia (17.7%), Solomon Islands (18.7%), Guam (21.5%), Mauritius (22%), French Polynesia (22.6%), Kiribati (22.7%), New Caledonia (23.4%), and the top, Nauru (24.1%). Why do Pacific Islanders have such high rates? The main reason is obesity. On the average, 50% are overweight, and on some islands, it is 90%. Women in American Samoa, for instance, are 80% obese. These islands are a territory of the USA. Imported fast foods and processed foods are the cause. In Fiji, only 16% of the population reaches 55 years and above. The rest all die early from non-communicable diseases. The people of these islands are literally eating themselves to death.

The reasons behind these huge differences have been of interest to scientists for some time, without any definitive answers. Clearly, there are genetic and environmental factors responsible. On these islands, the genetic make-up of these islanders is clearly not matched with the imported foods they are consuming. They would be better off going back to their traditional diet.

A comparison of Turkey and Azerbaijan is instructive. Both are ethnically similar and have similar genetic heritage. Their language is very similar. Turkey has a prevalence of 15%, and Azerbaijan has a rate of 2.6%. There probably is not much difference in exercise levels, as both cultures have many similarities. Here, I think the dietary factor may be the main difference. Whereas Turkish culinary culture has more carbs and sweet desserts, Azeris eat mainly barbecued meat, raw vegetables, and very little bread. The government organizes summer camps for diabetic children.

Both countries suffer from a massive obesity problem (32.1% in Turkey, and 29.1% in Azerbaijan).

Nevertheless, these differences are extremely difficult to isolate between one country and the next. Perhaps it may not be that productive to ponder these questions. After all, we can't do anything about our genes. On the other hand, we know a lot about how to modify lifestyle to either prevent diabetes or ameliorate its effects.

I think what is most important to realize is that the disease is a pandemic and is set to completely overload health systems. By 2050, one in three Americans will have diabetes. It will be the leading cause of new cases of blindness under the age of 75, and of kidney failure and non-injury amputations of the leg and foot, among adults.

Besides global warming, this may be one of the greatest threats to mankind. The sad thing is that most governments are at a loss as to how to deal with this. The UK government introduced a sugar tax, which is not a bad idea. The Singapore government came up with exhortations to diet and exercise, which of course is unlikely to make any impact whatsoever. Most governments are doing absolutely nothing to stem the tide.

Once you finish this book, you will realize that there are options to reverse the disease, which is another weapon we can use against this disease.

Next, we will talk about how diabetes can damage your body and lead to horrific consequences.

Chapter 2

What Can Diabetes Do to You?

Diabetes, until recently, was considered a lifelong, chronic, incurable disease, with a whole gamut of really bad sequelae. Industry and medical specialties grew up to manage this unsolvable problem, and this became a trillion dollar business. Diabetes can be a personal hell, especially for those with type 1 disease. It can seriously degrade health and lifestyle.

Diabetes mainly attacks blood vessels. It damages both small and large vessels. This leads to two quite distinct groups of diseases, although they can occasionally act in tandem.

Large Vessel Disease

Seventy-five percent of diabetics will die from a heart attack, and 16% will die from stroke. Diabetes damages large blood vessels by a process called atherosclerosis. Fatty deposits accumulate on the walls of large vessels, narrowing them and impeding blood supply to the target organs, much like road works impeding traffic on highways. The two most vulnerable organs are the heart and the brain.

For diabetics aged 65 years and above, 68% will die from heart disease, and 16% from stroke. Forty percent of patients with coronary artery disease have diabetes as a co-morbidity. Atherosclerotic disease prevalence in diabetics is 32.2%, and 21.2% have coronary artery disease.

Patients on insulin have another problem, which is a higher risk of complications when going for an angiogram to diagnose or treat their coronary artery disease.

If you require a coronary artery bypass operation, and you have diabetes, there is a 30% higher chance of dying from the procedure. So that's pretty bad news all around.

Next, we go to the legs. Twenty percent of diabetics have peripheral arterial disease. This leads to decreased blood supply, especially to the legs, which leads to pain when walking or climbing stairs, and eventually incapacitation. Ischemic legs are also prone to sores, and foot and leg infections that don't heal and may result in amputation. This disease is aggravated by nerve disease, also due to diabetes, which leads to loss of sensation and also poor healing of leg sores, ulcers, and wounds. One in 30 result in amputation. This is grim.

Small Vessel Disease

Diabetes has even more destructive potential when it comes to small vessels. High blood sugar literally wreaks havoc on the micro-circulation, and this has many effects, depending on where the destruction takes place.

Kidney

The kidney is the most vulnerable target. High blood sugar puts stress on the filtration system or glomeruli of the kidneys, which now has to filter through more water to wash out the sugar. Diabetes also often leads to hypertension, which is damaging to the kidneys. The first sign of trouble is usually albumin in the urine. This appears in small amounts in the beginning, and is termed microalbuminuria. In one study, 36.3% of diabetics had albumin in the urine.

What Can Diabetes Do to You?

Twenty to thirty percent of diabetics will go on to develop diabetic kidney disease, which is called diabetic nephropathy. Some of these will end up with end stage kidney failure and will need dialysis. A few lucky ones may get a transplant, but with ongoing diabetes, the new kidney may start to get damaged.

About 60% of patients on dialysis are there because of diabetic nephropathy. Diabetic nephropathy in early stages can be reversed if blood sugar is brought down promptly and permanently, and hypertension is controlled. This is best done by metabolic surgery. Prompt metabolic surgery, in patients already with early kidney disease, may save many patients from dialysis and transplantation.

Nerves

Diabetics get nerve problems because the disease attacks the microcirculation to the nerves, leading to nerve damage. This problem is worse in diabetics who are smokers. Diabetics often get loss of sensation, numbness, and tingling of the extremities. The distribution is classically glove and stocking. There may even be nerve pain from neuropathy. These symptoms are extremely difficult to treat medically, and are chronic and intractable.

Thirty to forty percent of diabetics suffer from nerve problems. Medical treatment to control the blood sugar may not reverse these nerve problems.

Diabetes may also affect the autonomic nervous system. This affects a host of systems, and produces many varied symptoms. It affects the heart rate and blood pressure, digestive system, bladder, sex organs, eyes, and ability to detect hypoglycemia. In the gastrointestinal tract, it can cause constipation, diarrhea, or both, and problems with swallowing and vomiting.

Autonomic neuropathy can accelerate aging and lead to sudden death from cardiac problems.

One of my patients, who was 40-plus years old, was a dog groomer. He ran his own business and was a leading brand in this exotic field. He was diabetic and was on 60 units of insulin a day, and he looked seventy. A gastric bypass cured his diabetes. His white hair turned black again, and he literally looked twenty years younger after his diabetes went into remission.

One of the commonest issues in diabetes is the diabetic foot. This is caused by poor circulation to the limbs, as well as to sensory neuropathy. Diabetics often have numbness of the toes and feet. Injuries and infections may go undetected and fester. If not attended to promptly, the infection spreads and can lead to gangrene and amputation.

Amputation

Let's talk a little more about this horrifying topic. Diabetes is the leading cause of leg and foot amputation. Eighty percent of non-traumatic amputations have their root in diabetes. Injuries and sores in diabetics occur and are neglected because there is no pain, as nerves are dead. Poor circulation results in delayed healing, and reduced resistance to infection may lead to infections in the feet and legs getting out of control and spreading. Tissues die and turn gangrenous.

What is less known is that after amputation, death soon follows. Diabetic amputees have a poor prognosis. Most die within 3 years. Amputation is a death sentence.

Not every diabetic foot infection leads to amputation: 60 to 80% heal, 10 to15% remain, and 5 to 24% end in amputation. The chance of saving a limb improves if the diabetes is reversed. The best way to reverse the diabetes quickly is by metabolic surgery.

Colonel L

This ex-military officer went on a trip to India and sustained a foot injury. He was a severe diabetic, on several different classes of medication, and already had neuropathy and microangiopathy. A large section of his foot and leg soon became gangrenous and turned black. He went through several rounds of surgical debridement of the dead tissue, and finally ended up with a skin graft.

The skin graft failed to take in several areas, and bone was exposed, which could not be covered. His orthopedic surgeon told him that if things didn't get better, an amputation was in the cards.

The Colonel was not obese and, in every other aspect, was healthy. His ability to walk was severely curtailed, and he could not exercise, which made his situation worse.

Even though he was not obese at that time, we had enough evidence that in the majority of patients, metabolic surgery would reverse diabetes, even in the low BMI. The Colonel was an athlete when he was younger.

The foremost thing that he wanted was to save his leg from amputation. He had read the grim statistics of death within years once that happened.

We checked him out and found that other than the diabetes and the rotting leg, he was reasonably healthy. We performed a modified RNY gastric bypass for him, leaving him a larger gastric pouch, as weight loss was not his prime objective. His recovery was uneventful, and his leg began to heal rapidly. He came off medication and could maintain normal blood sugars.

The effect on his healing and resistance to infection was remarkable. The skin graft on his leg began to look healthier, and the defects that exposed his bone began to close over.

In a few weeks, he was totally mobile again and could walk several kilometers all on his own.

His leg healed completely after 6 months, which was much more rapid than expected. His orthopedic surgeon gave him a prognosis of one year at least for the healing of his leg wounds and grafts.

The Colonel is happily back to work and his normal everyday activities. Metabolic surgery often has an amazing and unexpected effect on diabetic complications. Many a time, these complications are surprisingly reversed, or at least improved, after the surgery.

On the whole, 5 out of 1000 diabetics would end up with amputation.

Diabetes and the Eye

Diabetic eye disease is one of the major causes of blindness. Diabetes damages the microcirculation of the retina of the eye, leading to exudates and hemorrhages. The disease is called diabetic retinopathy and is progressive and can lead to blindness. Treatment requires laser and surgery. One percent to 1.3% of diabetics will go blind from this problem.

Forty percent of diabetics will get some degree of diabetic retinopathy. This emphasizes the need for diabetics to go for a retinal scan regularly. Actually, this rule probably applies to everyone. When caught early, there is effective treatment; if discovered late, the condition may be irreversible.

Once again, metabolic surgery can have a surprisingly significant effect in reversing this condition and improving the eyesight of patients. The problem is microangiopathy or damage to the small blood vessels. Reversing the diabetes will stop the damage and allow time for repair and healing. Many patients have reported clear vision after surgery.

Sexual Problems in Diabetics

Male diabetics experience erectile dysfunction (ED). One study shows that 50% of diabetic men have ED, which is 3.5 times the prevalence in controls. 12.3% have mild ED, 30.9% have mild to moderate, 19.1% have moderate, and 16.4% have severe ED.

Erectile dysfunction occurs because diabetes affects both the circulation as well as the innervation of the penis. It may be one of the manifestations of autonomic neuropathy, which has a wide range of manifestations.

Many diabetic men wake up in the morning with no morning erection. Medical control of the blood sugar may not help this condition. Metabolic surgery may help this problem.

It is also quite surprising how many female diabetics are affected by sexual dysfunction related to their diabetes.

The prevalence of sexual dysfunction was 78.7%. Among these, 58% reported problems in lubrication, 50% complained of decreased sexual desire, 50% had problems with arousal, 47.3% had dyspareunia, 32.7% complained of orgasmic dysfunction, and 42.7% reported problems in sexual satisfaction.

One of my patients was a middle-aged engineer in her 50s, who had moderate to severe diabetes and a diabetic foot problem. Her doctor gave her a grim prognosis of having to face amputation at some point. She and her husband had not much of a sex life, as he had medical issues as well.

After metabolic surgery, Ms. T was completely reversed with normal blood sugars, and she came off all medication. Her leg also got better and very swiftly healed and became normal except for dry skin. She went back to work and became very active, climbing the hill behind her apartment block every morning.

Unfortunately, her husband died in his sleep just 3 months after her surgery. Ms. T experienced an overwhelming increase in sexual desire and libido, and being a conservative woman, had no outlet for her needs.

Casual sex didn't appeal to her, and she sought a long-term, exclusive relationship, which at her age wasn't going to be found easily. Finally, she migrated to a different country, seeking greener pastures.

I guess curing a disease can sometimes also bring some unforeseen consequences!

Skin Problems in Diabetes

Diabetes is also associated with a host of skin problems. Sometimes general physicians and dermatologists forget to check for diabetes when they see these problems, and they treat them topically with creams and other application medicine, which usually does not solve the problem.

Scleroderma diabeticorum is a rare condition affecting type 2 diabetics. It causes thickening of the skin on the back of the neck and upper back. Although moisturizers may help, the best treatment is to bring the blood sugar down, either by medicine or surgery.

Both type 1 and type 2 diabetes can cause ugly hypopigmented patches, called vitiligo. The cells that make pigment in the skin are destroyed. Treatment may require tattooing of the affected areas, as the discoloration is permanent.

What Can Diabetes Do to You?

Acanthosis nigricans results in darkening and thickening of the skin, especially in the skin folds. It precedes diabetes and strikes people who are overweight. It is a manifestation of insulin resistance. Losing weight may help and, of course, reversing the diabetes.

Atherosclerosis reduces blood supply to the affected area and can result in skin changes, especially in the lower limbs, such as hair loss, thinning of the skin, shiny skin, cold skin, and discolored toe nails. This may presage developing foot and leg infections, the so-called diabetic foot syndrome.

Necrobiosis lipoidica diabeticorum sounds exotically Latin. This is caused by changes in the fat and collagen under the skin. The skin becomes thin and reddened, and ulcerates easily. Again, this is a precursor of diabetic foot and leg infections, which can progress to gangrene and amputation. Any sores must be attended to promptly. Diabetic dermapathy are called shin spots. They are due to damage to blood vessels in the skin, and appear as shiny round or oval patches on the front of the lower leg. They may be itchy or have a burning sensation.

Digital sclerosis affects the fingers and toes, and makes the skin thick, waxy, and tight. Treatment is diabetic control.

Eruptive xanthamatosis appears as yellow, waxy, pea-like bumps on the skin of the face and buttocks, back of the arms and legs, and in the creases. They occur because of difficulty in clearing fat. Diabetics often have high triglycerides in the blood, and this can also lead to pancreatitis. Fat lowering medication may be necessary.

There are a host of other skin problems, including rashes and blisters. In bullosis diabeticorum, blisters occur on fingers, toes, hands, feet, legs, and forearms. Luckily, they heal on their own. They happen in poorly controlled diabetes, and in those with diabetic neuropathy.

Disseminated granuloma annulare are ring or arc shaped lesions, occurring on the fingers, ears, chest, and abdomen. They can be red, red-brown, or skin colored. Steroids, like hydrocortisone, may help.

In addition, diabetics are prone to a host of bacterial and fungal infections of the skin, due to reduced resistance to infection.

The take-home message here is that if you have skin problems, don't forget to check your blood or urine sugar. Diabetes could be the underlying cause, and reversing the diabetes may solve the problem. Sometimes your GP or dermatologist may forget that and have to be reminded.

Diabetic Ketoacidosis

In this condition, the blood sugar gets very high, and your body then produces blood acids called ketones. Your body is breaking down fat as fuel because there is not enough insulin to drive sugar into cells. The blood then becomes acidotic. There are symptoms of extreme thirst, nausea and vomiting, abdominal pain, and confusion. There are ketones in the breath and in the urine. Eventually, the patient will go into a coma, and death will follow unless the condition is promptly managed and reversed. It mainly occurs in type 1 diabetes but can happen to poorly controlled type 2 as well.

Looking at how damaging diabetes is, it would be obvious to you that reversing or curing the disease could be one of the best decisions you are ever going to make in your life.

Remember that medical treatment cannot cure your disease. Strict lifestyle changes can control your disease but have to be kept up lifelong. It isn't easy. The easiest way to solve the problem is metabolic surgery.

Chapter 3

What Are the Types of Diabetes, and What Are Their Causes?

Most people are aware that there are two types of diabetes: type 1 and type 2. Type 1 diabetics produce almost no insulin and, therefore, are totally insulin dependent. Type 2 diabetics may or may not need insulin. Both conditions are known to be dangerous and life threatening.

Today, we know that this subject is more complex than most non-medical people think. Let's discuss the various types of diabetes mellitus.

Type 1 Diabetes

This is also known as juvenile diabetes, or insulin-dependent diabetes. The exact cause still remains a mystery, but it is largely thought to be autoimmune. Genetics and viruses are also possible causes. In this disease, there is a total shutdown of insulin production by the beta cells of the pancreas. These patients are insulin dependent and will die without the insulin injections.

They suffer from the standard symptoms of diabetes, such as thirst and frequent urination, and may have unexplained weight loss. They are at high risk of ketoacidosis and coma.

Despite some promising research on stem cells, there is yet to be a reliable way to resolve this disease. Surgical options include islet cells or pancreatic organ transplant, but this would lead to a lifelong dependence on immune suppression, which would be as deleterious as, or worse than, being on insulin.

Fortunately, only 5% of diabetics are of this type. It can start in childhood, but adults can develop this disease as well.

At the moment, these patients are condemned to a life of insulin injections in one form or another. There is still no good solution for type 1. Researchers are working on stem cells but, to date, no one has been able to find a way to induce stem cells to differentiate in islet cells, which produce insulin. Giving undifferentiated stem cells is a hit-or-miss treatment. It sometimes works, but the success rate is low and short lived. It's also very expensive and has to be repeated to sustain any effect it might have. I seriously doubt that this is a worthwhile option for many.

These patients are subject to all the problems of being insulin dependent, and need to inject themselves multiple times every single day. Unless they have one of those blood sugar devices attached to their skin, they also need to constantly check their blood sugar, several times a day, which means more pricks.

Type 1 diabetics' whole lives revolve around their blood sugar levels. Every bit of activity or consumption affects it. They have to constantly decide how much insulin to give themselves—too much, and they go hypoglycemic; too little, and the blood sugar spikes.

The only surgery that works is either islet cell transplant or whole organ pancreatic transplant. This is usually done in conjunction with a kidney transplant, for kidney failure resulting from diabetes. This still condemns the patient to a life of drugs. From then on, it's immunosuppressants, which is also miserable and lifelong. A double transplant is a major undertaking and is not often done unless the patient happens to be very fortunate and gets a donor. Otherwise, it's a combination of insulin and dialysis, which is then doubly miserable. The main advantage is, of course, to get off kidney dialysis.

What about metabolic or bariatric surgery for type 1 diabetics? Some cases have been done in Cleveland Clinic, and they have recorded some benefit in terms of easier control and less insulin requirements, as the main idea is to reduce insulin resistance by correcting the obesity. The patient will still require insulin but will benefit hugely from the weight loss.

Uncommonly, there is a type 1b diabetes, which has complete insulin deficiency, with no evidence of autoimmunity. It has a strong genetic basis.

Type 2 Diabetes

This comprises the vast majority of diabetics. The statistics vary with each country, but on the average, 95% of diabetics are type 2. In China, maybe only 1 in 100,000 are type 1, but in Scandinavia, for instance, type 1 incidence may be 20 in 10,000.

Type 2 diabetes generally occurs after 40 years of age, but I have seen 13-year-old type 2s. So age is a general guideline, but there are always exceptions. Similarly, type 1 can occur in older people, though most start when pretty young.

I saw a 13-year-old boy in Qatar, who turned out to be type 2 even though he got diabetes when young. He was obese. A sleeve resection immediately put him back to a non-diabetic state.

In type 2, there is either insulin deficiency, insulin resistance, or both. The causation is multifactorial, and there are genes involved, but the lifestyle and environment plays a big part. In the USA, 85% of diabetics are fat, and the obesity leads to insulin resistance, which causes the diabetes. Nevertheless, if you have close family members with type 2 diabetes, you have a higher chance of getting the disease.

When you measure the C peptide in these patients, which is an index of endogenous insulin production, type 2 diabetics usually exhibit a normal or high C peptide, showing that they still have a good capacity to produce insulin. The insulin level is high because they have insulin resistance, which forces the islet cells to produce higher levels of insulin to overcome the resistance.

Type 2 diabetes shows a wide range of severity: from very mild, which is controllable by diet and exercise; to moderate, which requires oral medication; to severe, which requires insulin. However, all of them have some degree of increased insulin resistance.

Until recently, there was thought to be no cure for type 2s. Diet and exercise can control the mildest cases, but this has to be sustained lifelong; and as the patient ages, the diabetes usually gets worse, and may require medication. Most type 2 diabetics are on oral medication, and most are maintained this way for life.

Up to 50% of type 2s eventually deteriorate enough to get on insulin, and thus have to live a life like that of the type 1s. Although the diabetes in type 2, on the whole, is not as severe as type one, there is a statistical reduction of life expectancy by at least 10 years. Most type 2s will die of a heart attack or a stroke, or develop cancer.

The really good news is that most type 2 diabetics can be reversed or even cured by metabolic surgery.

Until recently, when you Googled the question, "Can diabetes be cured?" you would get the standard answer: "There is no cure for diabetes. Diet and exercise may help to keep the blood sugar under control." This was also the standard teaching and belief in the medical community.

What Are the Types of Diabetes, and What Are Their Causes?

Recently, when I did an internet search, I was pleasantly surprised to read this:

Permanent Cure for Diabetes

Yes – It can be cured permanently by metabolic and bariatric surgery. Till about a few years ago, there was **no permanent cure** for diabetes. However, new research finds that diabetes is a *curable disease*.

Actually, this is not entirely accurate, as metabolic surgery has already been around for 20 years. There are scientific publications going way back, which clearly demonstrates this. In 2016, the American Diabetic Association put out a consensus statement that clearly recognizes surgery as an equivalent option to medical treatment.

Gestational Diabetes

Two to five percent of women will get diabetes during pregnancy, and this happens usually around the 24th to the 28th week. This condition will require close follow-up by the obstetrician, and can most times be managed by a diet and exercise program, but it may sometimes require drugs or insulin. During pregnancy, one has to avoid medication if possible, to avoid unknown effects on the fetus.

Most times, the condition resolves after delivery, but the woman is at much higher risk of developing diabetes later in life, and this happens in 50% of cases.

It is prudent for women with this condition to regularly check their fasting blood sugar levels and HbA1c, and to remain vigilant for life.

MODY: Maturity Onset Diabetes of the Young

This only occurs in 1 to 2% of diabetics. Some estimate the incidence to be up to 5%. In these cases, the diabetes is caused by a single gene, which nowadays can be detected by gene testing. In this disease, a single gene mutation disrupts insulin production. Despite the name, it can occur at any age. Those that happen in the young can mislead doctors to assume that it is type 1, and consign the patient to lifelong insulin. Many types of MODY, however, can have a better outcome, and some can even be reversed. The severity is variable and depends on the gene affected.

There are now 11 types of MODY. Each is designated by a single gene. They range in severity from mild to those requiring insulin. MODY 1, 3, and 4 can be managed with medication called sulphonylureas. MODY 2 can be treated with diet and exercise. It is probably the mildest variety, though having this gene could cause some problems in pregnancy. MODY 1 can sometimes degenerate and require insulin. MODY 5 and 6 require insulin. MODY 6 is associated with kidney cysts. MODY 7 to eleven are newly discovered varieties.

This potential for metabolic surgery in this field has not been studied well, because these types of diabetes are rare. The other thing is that most MODY patients are lean. I expect that the milder forms of the disease, in those who are fat, may be amenable to metabolic surgery, which would get them off sulphonylureas.

LADA: Latent Autoimmune Diabetes of Adulthood – Type 1.5

This occurs in 10 to 25% of diabetics. In this condition, the body also stops producing insulin, just like type 1 diabetes. The progression, however, is much slower. Very often, the patient appears to be type 2, but gradually, the diabetes gets worse, and the patient eventually requires insulin and becomes just like a type 1. Some endocrinologists label this condition as type 1.5 diabetes.

In 10% of individuals, this occurs over 35 years of age; and in 25%, it occurs at a younger age group.

What Are the Types of Diabetes, and What Are Their Causes?

These patients typically have antibodies in the blood, which can help with the diagnosis. It must be suspected if diabetes status suddenly starts deteriorating.

This condition is most disappointing when it occurs after metabolic surgery. I had one patient from Malaysia who made a very good recovery after a gastric bypass, and successfully got off all medication. Then, within months, his blood sugar started to climb again. We were really shocked by this.

Checking his anti-islet cell and anti-GAD antibodies showed the cause. His C peptide also showed a steep decline. He had developed LADA and was transitioning to become like a type 1 diabetic. He went back on insulin, and we could not offer him much.

From then on, if the C peptide was low, we would usually check for antibodies so that we don't operate on someone who has LADA or is developing LADA.

I think that many of the failures of metabolic surgery in diabetes may be due to this condition. If we screen out these cases, the success rate for metabolic surgery would remain very high.

There are a few very rare types of diabetes.

Neonatal Diabetes Mellitus

This is diabetes that occurs in infants before 6 months of age. It can happen anywhere between birth and 6 months. It is a monogenic disease and occurs in one in 100,000, to one in 500,000, live births. There are two varieties. One is transient and disappears but may reappear later in life; the other is permanent. It is often mistaken as type 1 diabetes, which usually occurs at less than 6 months of age.

Type 3 Diabetes

Diabetes is not only about high blood sugar; it causes inflammation throughout the body. Therefore, diabetics have a much higher risk of heart disease and Alzheimer's disease. Alzheimer's disease can now be considered type 3 diabetes. Insulin resistance and insulin growth factor are a key part of Alzheimer's disease. Type 2 diabetics have a 50% to 65% increased risk of developing Alzheimer's disease. This information was gleaned from the National Center for Health Statistics.

Chapter 4

Wish List for Those with Type 2 Diabetes

Most diabetics have a long wish list. They look to their doctors to achieve these goals, but most times, these expectations are not met. Here are the usual items on the list, and you can see that it is quite long.

- Maintain normal fasting blood sugar
- Get off insulin
- Get off oral antidiabetic medication
- Eat whatever I like
- Take sugar, carbohydrates, and desserts
- Reverse hypertension and get off pills
- Reverse high cholesterol and get off pills
- Reverse fatty liver
- Live longer
- Reduce chance of getting cancer
- Reduce chance of getting heart disease and stroke
- Save legs
- Reverse nerve problems that cause pain, numbness, and tingling
- Save eyes
- Save kidneys
- Lose weight
- Get pregnant
- Improve sexual drive and function
- Improve wound healing
- Improve resistance to infection

- Improve physical fitness
- Save on time spent seeing doctors and going to hospital
- Spend less on health

This would be a typical wish list of many diabetic patients. In an ideal world, we would be able to grant all these myriad of wishes. The amazing thing is that we actually can, with present technology.

Most of these goals are not achievable by conventional treatment, which is medicine, injections, and lifestyle changes. Conventional treatment can bring down your blood sugar but does not address the primary disease. Most drugs also do not reduce cardiovascular and cancer risk. Certainly, diabetics will lose at least 10 years of life expectancy, even with conventional management.

For years, I have Googled: "Cure for Diabetes Mellitus." For years, it has come back with the answer: "There is no cure for diabetes mellitus, but lifestyle changes may bring the condition under control in some cases." This occurred whether I used Google or Internet Explorer.

If you look at the wish list above, every item on the wish list can be fulfilled by metabolic surgery, except one.

Guess!

Yes, you are right—you can't eat whatever you like. The cure is dependent on having a reasonably healthy diet. You still need to reduce your carbohydrate intake, and minimize your intake of sugar. You still need to watch your portions. Unrestricted diet and weight gain will lead to recurrence. Do not revert to old, bad habits. Learn to live a healthy lifestyle.

You will reap all the other 22 benefits. There are so many true life stories of remarkable recoveries that it would fill many books.

Wish List for Those with Type 2 Diabetes

"C" was a rather pretty but young, obese Singaporean lady who had polycystic ovarian disease (PCOS) and diabetes. She had trouble conceiving. She had a sleeve resection. After surgery, she slimmed down significantly and became even prettier, and her diabetes resolved. Her periods became regular and, after a year, she conceived. Recently, she gave birth to a beautiful baby. Resolving her weight and diabetes problems improved her fertility and made this possible. I now tell ladies with PCOS that one of the best solutions to the problem is metabolic or bariatric surgery.

Hypertension and High Cholesterol

Metabolic surgery can reverse both of these pretty effectively. Hypertension usually disappears as quickly as the diabetes, and high cholesterol usually comes down in months, to usually normal levels in a year. If the patient is obese and hypertensive, that is enough to justify the operation—to get him back to a normal blood pressure, free from hypertensive drugs. Indeed, metabolic surgery is also a cure for high blood pressure. This is another disease thought to be incurable.

Diabetic Kidney Disease

Metabolic surgery is considered the best treatment for diabetic kidney disease. The kidney problem can be arrested or even reversed. I have seen albumin in the urine disappear, kidney function improve, and patients saved from dialysis once their diabetes is reversed.

Fatty Liver

Fatty liver invariably improves after metabolic surgery. Patients may be saved a future liver transplant if they have surgery early enough.

Diabetic Retinopathy

Diabetes causes haemorrhage and exudates in the retina of the eye, causing blurring of vision. If left to progress, this leads to blindness. Metabolic surgery improves the condition almost immediately. Very often, the patients have clear vision after their diabetes is reversed. This effect is often very prompt.

Neuropathy

Diabetics can have pain, numbness, tingling, and other nerve symptoms due to diabetic nerve disease. After surgery, these conditions frequently reverse as well. The neuropathy can lead to sores and ulcers that do not heal. These can become infected and lead to gangrene and amputation. Reversing the neuropathy can thus be limb saving.

Effect on Large Vessel Disease

Metabolic surgery is less successful in reversing large vessel complications like coronary artery disease and cerebrovascular disease. Once plaques are formed inside vessels, reversing diabetes may not make them go away. Reversing diabetes does slow down the development of these lesions, however. Vessel disease is due to inflammation, and diabetes causes inflammation. Reversing the diabetes reduces the inflammation.

Sexual Disorders Due to Diabetes

Most diabetic men have erectile dysfunction. This can improve once the diabetes is reversed. Women also have sexual dysfunction, the most common being a loss of libido. This can surprisingly return strongly once the diabetes is reversed. As illustrated in the story above, fertility issues also tend to resolve, and women often conceive after surgery.

Wish List for Those with Type 2 Diabetes

In summary, there are a host of benefits to be reaped from reversing diabetes with surgery, as the downstream sequelae and complications of diabetes often get better and may resolve.

Chapter 5

Controlling Diabetes by Lifestyle Management

I am asked this question a lot. Every diabetic wants to know if he or she can go it alone, without expensive and inconvenient medical intervention. Well, the short answer is yes. You can control type 2 diabetes by having a very strict and rigorous lifestyle regime. This is especially so if you are overweight or obese, and if your diabetes is not too severe. The caveat is that it is pretty damn hard. You would have to display the discipline of a Navy SEAL.

The good news is that in Western countries, 30% of obese people have diabetes, and 85% of diabetics are fat. The overweight or obese diabetic has the best chance of controlling, or even reversing, their diabetes by self-control. All you have to do is stop eating! Most of you won't be able to do that for long.

In Asia, the situation is somewhat different. Diabetics are generally thinner but have more visceral fat, and exercise much less. Compared to Caucasians, Asians have 3 to 5% more body fat for the same BMI. Caucasians with a BMI of 30 have a body fat percentage of 25% in young adult males, and 35% in young adult females. Chinese males with a BMI of 23.7 have 25% body fat, and females with a BMI of 21.2 have 32% body fat.

If you are fortunate enough to be an overweight or obese type 2 diabetic, your best strategy is to lose weight by any means you can.

Here are some areas of your life that you must pay attention to if you want to control your diabetes purely by lifestyle changes. You can also institute the same changes even if you are on drug management, and it would improve your control.

Give up sugar

The consumption of large amounts of sugar is one of the main causes of the increased incidence of diabetes. Much of our food is unnecessarily sweet. Soft drinks and sodas are a major offender. Desserts and ice cream are also deleterious. In some countries, there is a plethora of sweet desserts, which are consumed on a daily basis. In my travels, I noticed this most in Turkey, Azerbaijan, India, and Indonesia. The USA, Australia, and most Western countries are also guilty. I only need to point to the sumptuous desserts in cities like Vienna. They are sinfully deliciously but can be ultimately deadly.

Switching to artificial sweeteners is a possible option, but the latest scientific data seems to show that they may be harmful; and they certainly do not seem to result in any loss of weight or improvement in diabetes. I seem to see more and more articles on this subject. The more definitive step would be to give up your passion for sweets altogether. Actually, if you avoid sweets for a while, you will lose the taste for them. Diabetics should take a dessert only once a month, or at most, once a fortnight.

Typically, if you are serious about dietary sugars, you should give it up as completely as you can. That means no sugar in coffee or tea, no desserts, and no sweeteners. In Asia, some things you should look out for, in regard to sugar, are the ingredients in sauces. An example is sweet black soya sauce, known as *kecap manis* in Indonesia and Malaysia. It is also used on chicken rice in Singapore. Sweet peanut sauce, used as a garnish for meat skewers, or satay, is also another often overlooked item.

Sugar is used everywhere in most processed foods. It is present in cakes, bread, pastries, biscuits, and nearly everything people normally eat. If you are determined to control your diabetes by diet, then you must be super alert and super aware.

Cut down drastically on carbohydrates

The next thing you have to give up are carbohydrates. Carbohydrates are a large part of any diet and are really difficult to reduce. It's present in rice, bread, cakes, pasta, noodles, potatoes, and starchy root vegetables. Carbohydrates are the staple in most diets across cultures. In Asia, the main problem is white rice. Almost all cultures here take it in huge quantities, and this is the main cause of the alarming rise in diabetes incidence in Asia. Here, many cultures eat rice three times a day. Even breakfast is rice. In Malaysia and Indonesia, natives eat a breakfast of coconut rice, called *Nasi Lemak*. In Chinese culture, rice porridge is a common breakfast food. Rice may be the main cause of the diabetes epidemic in the East.

The highest diabetes incidence is in the Middle East. Saudi Arabia has 20.2%, Kuwait 17.8%, Bahrain 17.3%, and Qatar, 15.7%. East Asia is better in terms of percentages but worse because of far larger populations. Malaysia has 10.1% diabetics, China 11.5% (113.9 million people), and India, 7.1% (62 million people). Indonesia has about 7%, and also has a huge population of 250 million people. All these countries are rice eating.

To have an effective antidiabetic diet, you have to eat a minimum of rice, and what you eat should be brown or unpolished rice. Basmati rice is also a variety that has a relatively low glycemic index. To reduce the elevation of blood sugar, it is best to eat rice only with fibre or fat, to delay absorption. It is found, for example, that Singaporean chicken rice, which is white rice coated in chicken fat, has a better glycemic index than plain white rice.

Processed flour is the other concern. Most bread products, pastries, and cakes are made from processed white wheat flour, which has a high glycemic index and leaches quickly in the blood stream as sugar. Brown breads and high fibre breads are safer to eat, as the fibre prevents the rapid absorption of the starch, and there is a lower rise in sugar after consuming them. On an anti-diabetic diet, it is best to avoid all white bread, or any product made from processed white flour. Indian breads are also an interesting subject. They are no doubt seriously delicious. Most have a high glycemic index, so the best are roti or chapatti, made from whole grain or cracked wheat. One of the worst things for a diabetic to eat is a doughnut.

The other heavily consumed carbohydrate product is potatoes. Potatoes can have a variable effect on blood sugar, depending on the type of potato, the ripeness of the potato, and how it is cooked. Boiling potatoes with the skin on is probably the best way to cook them, in terms of keeping blood sugar low. Potatoes also have a lower glycemic index when consumed cold rather than hot. Microwaved and mashed potatoes have the highest glycemic index, so diabetics should avoid eating potatoes that way. French fries are moderate. Please remember that quantity also matters, so taking large quantities would negate all the care you take keeping the glycemic index low, because the total carbohydrate load will be high.

Pasta and noodles are also foods to avoid. If you need a carbohydrate fix, you should limit it to once a day, small portions, and never in the evening or night. Concerning pasta, boiling the pasta too long increases the glycemic index. Macaroni and cheese is the worse pasta dish. Fettuccini, eaten al dente, with minimal cooking, probably has the lowest glycemic index. Whole grain pasta also has a lower glycemic index, in the moderate range.

Chinese wheat noodles have a glycemic index of 82, which is high. Japanese soba noodles, which are made from buckwheat (glycemic index 59), have a low glycemic load as well. One cup of soba has 25g of carbohydrates, and a glycemic load of only 9. This is assuming that the soba is real buckwheat and not adulterated with normal flour. Udon noodles also have a low glycemic index (53). Here again, you should avoid overcooking, and eat the soba cold.

What is the best grain? The best grain for a diabetic to eat is barley, which has the lowest glycemic index. I am sure that you can look up some nice barley recipes to assuage your carbohydrate craving.

In summary, if you are diabetic and you need to control your carbohydrates, then it is best to restrict them to only one portion a day, and have it for lunch or breakfast. You also need to watch the portion size and the glycemic index and load of your carbohydrate fix for the day. Choose low glycemic index options whenever you can. Never eat carbs at night.

The Controversial Subject of Fruits and Fruit Juice

We all love fruits, so it is hard to give them up just because one has diabetes. Besides, fruits have so many vitamins and phytochemicals that are good for you. Unfortunately, fruits all contain sugar, and too much fruit is bad for your diabetes.

When considering which fruits to eat, it is more useful to consider the glycemic load rather than the glycemic index. A good example is watermelon. This fruit has a glycemic index of 72, which is high. The sugar in this fruit comes out immediately into the bloodstream. Interestingly though, the quantity per portion of carbohydrate in this fruit is low, so the glycemic load per 120g portion is only 4, which is relatively low.

A good site to check out the glycemic load of various fruits is: https://adrenalfatiguesolution.com/fruits-lowest-glycemic-load/

The best fruits, with the lowest glycemic index, are limes and strawberries, with a GL of 1/120g; and apricots, grapefruits, and lemons, at 3/120g. Moderately good ones are guava, nectarines, oranges, and pears, at 4/120g. Terrible fruits are mangos at 8g, cherries at 9g, prunes at 10g, and bananas at 11g. If you really like these fruits, eat small portions only.

Even worse are figs, dates, and raisins, at 16, 18, and 28. It's best not to go anywhere near raisins.

How much fruit then, per day? The recommendation is no more than 2 portions, and never at dinner or after dinner. At least, you should give your body a chance to burn off the sugar during the day when you are active.

In summary, a diabetic wanting to keep their blood sugar under control, must limit fruit intake. They must also consider the glycemic index and load in the choice of fruits, and the timing of eating them. The best policy is to eat them for lunch and dinner only, have no more than two, 120-gram portions, and choose the ones with a low glycemic index and a low glycemic load. Eat more strawberries!

Let's now look at something more interesting. What are the foods that have the least calories per 100 grams?

Food with the Lowest Calories:
http://www.healthassist.net/food/calories-chart.shtml

Everything you eat or drink, besides plain water, contains calories. So what foods should you eat if you want to lose weight as well as keep diabetes in check?

Most of the lowest calorie foods are vegetables, but even here, there is a wide range: from watercress, which is 11 Kcal per 100 grams, to Brussels sprouts at 43 Kcal, beets at 44 kcal, broad beans at 72 Kcal, and finally, fava beans, at 88Kcal per 100 grams. It doesn't mean that you should avoid the beans, because they are also very high in protein. For ease of memory, let's divide vegetables up into high calorie, moderate calorie, and low calorie. Let's approach them in the reverse order.

Low calorie vegetables are those that have 20Kcal per 100 grams or below. Diabetics should really concentrate on eating these. They can fill you up without contributing too many fattening calories. If you stick to these vegetables alone, you can already have a varied and diverse meal repertoire. All of the ones below have about a glycemic index of 15, and are therefore considered low GI.

The lowest calorie vegetables are artichokes, asparagus, broccoli, cauliflower, eggplant, cucumber, green beans, lettuce, peppers, snow peas, spinach, young summer squash, and tomatoes. Most of these are the ingredients of the Mediterranean diet, which as everyone knows, is one of the healthiest, minus the pasta and pizza.

Is It Better to Be a Vegetarian?

This is a somewhat controversial question. Firstly, it is not necessary to be a vegetarian to control your diabetes by diet. Taking animal protein actually has the advantage of allowing one to eat less volume to maintain nutrition. The problem with vegetarians is that some tend to fill up the gaps by taking large amount of carbohydrates. This is a big disadvantage, as carbohydrates will not be good for the blood sugar levels.

On the other hand, it is definitely possible to be a vegetarian and still manage your diabetes. You will really have to watch your carbohydrate intake, and eat lots of vegetables. It is also good to take a lot of plant protein, like beans and soya, to maintain adequate protein intake.

Being vegetarian is better than being vegan. If vegetarians can eat eggs and dairy, there is usually no problem. Vegans, who do not even eat eggs or dairy, will need to consume large amounts of plant proteins, and this may pose some difficulty for some.

The answer to the original question is no. There is no advantage to being diabetic and vegetarian.

How Do I Manage Meat, Poultry, Fish, and Seafood?

The best animal protein is probably fish. It has Omega 3 and is probably the healthiest way to consume animal protein. There is one problem, though. Pollution of our seas, rivers, and lakes has led to the contamination of fish, etc., with heavy metals, notably mercury. The higher up the food chain, the heavier the contamination. The fish with the highest Hg content are:

- Grouper
- Chilean sea bass
- Bluefish
- Halibut
- Sablefish (black cod)
- Spanish mackerel (Gulf)
- Fresh tuna (except skipjack)
- Swordfish

The fish with the lowest levels of mercury are: salmon, tilapia, shrimp, tuna (canned light), cod, and catfish.

You can see that tuna appears twice. That is because the type of tuna is important. Albacore tuna or white tuna has high mercury, and skipjack tuna, used in canned light tuna, has low mercury levels.

The recommendation is at least two servings of fish a week, but there is no objection to eating fish daily, except that higher consumption doesn't lead to any better result. Pregnant women, however, should be careful about consuming too much fish, because of the mercury content.

How Safe Is Meat?

The good news is that there is no glycemic index for meat. That is because meat is protein and not carbohydrate. From the glycemic effect point of view alone, it is thus totally safe for the diabetic to eat meat.

Like in everything else about the food, the issues are far more complicated. Meat contains fat and cholesterol. Some meats are contaminated with hormones and antibiotics.

The very healthiest meat is actually lean pork tenderloin. A 100 gm serving has just 122 calories. I know, it's not a great choice for those who need halal or kosher meals, so millions of people won't eat it. Buffalo is the next, as it has less calories and fat than beef. The fat content is about half of that in beef. Some of the lesser known meats, which are particularly healthy, are ostrich and pheasant. Ostrich has half the fat content of chicken, and tastes like red meat even though it is not. These meats have low fat and high protein, and are not contaminated, unlike the more standard items.

Beef is good, but it depends on the type of beef. It is best to eat grass-fed beef from Argentina, Australia, or New Zealand. The grain-fed variety is less healthy because of the higher fat content, and also because of the contaminants in the grain. Chicken is a healthy meat, but commercial chicken has antibiotics and hormones. Otherwise, it is a really healthy choice. Most of the fat is in the skin, so it is best to eat it skinless. I know, the tastiest bits are the skin, especially when roasted and crispy. On the other hand, if you are diabetic and not overweight or obese, you can be less circumspect about consuming a little chicken skin.

Veal is also a good choice, with about 150 Kcal per 3 oz serving. It's not exactly cheap, and some people may object to slaughtering baby cattle, but it tastes really good and is quite healthy if the right cuts are chosen.

The meats to avoid are all the preserved ones, which all have either high sodium or high nitrates. The meats to avoid, or at least cut down on, include ham (high fat), prosciutto, corned beef, bacon, salami, mortadella, and hot dogs. The last is high in nitrates. Chicken nuggets are a disaster, as there is very little chicken, and it comes from all the worst parts of the animal. It is best not to feed it to your kids!

What about duck and goose? The problem with these birds is the high fat content, especially in the layer under the skin. Otherwise, the calorie content is not too disastrous, and goose is a somewhat lower in calories than duck. It is recommended that these birds be eaten in the nude, or minus skin. Where is the fun in that? The best and most delicious part of these birds is the skin, roasted to crispy perfection. If you are diabetic but have no weight issue, then go ahead and enjoy your Peking duck. What you really have to look out for is the sweet sauce that goes with it. Eaten Chinese style, the sauce may cause more problems than the duck or goose. Roasted German style may be healthier, with chestnuts and red kraut, and bathed in its own juices.

Alcohol

Alcoholic beverages, like beer and wine, contain calories, and if you are diabetic, and really must drink, then you should confine yourself to only one glass of wine or a half pint of beer.

Sodas and Other Sweet Drinks

These must be strictly avoided. They contain loads of sugar and have a very high glycemic index. Fruit juice from a carton, can, or bottle is also full of sugar and is in the same category. If you must drink fruit juice, have it freshly squeezed; or better still, just eat the fruit.

At this point, you have probably come to the conclusion that you have information overload, so why don't we summarize what a diabetic must do to keep the blood sugar in check with dietary control.

Firstly, you must watch the portions. In Western culture, the portions are usually at least 2 to 3 times too large. Eat half to one-third the amount you normally consume.

Secondly, watch the calorie content and glycemic index of the food you eat. Choose low glycemic index, low glycemic load, or both. Choose lower calorie alternatives, especially if you need to lose weight to improve your diabetes.

Stick to protein and vegetables. Meat, fish, poultry, and dairy are all fine.

Cut the carbohydrates, and choose low GI varieties.

Exercise

This is a crucial element. If you are diabetic, you should do 150 minutes a week of moderate exercise. This is the minimum. The exercise should take you to 60 to 70% of your maximum capacity, and no more. If you go all out, your blood sugar might actually rise, as adrenaline will be secreted. It is far better to go for a slow, steady burn. For a really fast effect on your blood sugar, it is recommended to do at least 30 minutes daily.

Another interesting finding is that just 15 minutes of brisk walking, after every meal, may lower your blood sugar by as much as 10 to 15%. Anyway, some exercise is always better than no exercise.

Physical activity is very much affected by culture, geography, and weather. Surprisingly, the most inactive country in the world is Malta! Saudi Arabia and Swaziland come second and third. I believe weather could be the cause. It's easier to do outdoor sports when the weather is nice or even cold.

In Southeast Asia, Malaysia tops the inactive list, and Indonesia is also rather indolent. There is also the factor of the exercise culture; in some countries, this is well developed, and in others, it is not. In Jakarta, for instance, the terrible traffic, with massive traffic jams, makes it almost impossible to cycle on the streets or even to take a healthy walk in the smog. Nevertheless, if you are diabetic, you need to make some effort to exercise.

Singapore has a good exercise culture, partly as a result of compulsory military service. After the 2 years in the army, all males are subjected to a rigorous physical fitness assessment, twice yearly, with penalties for not passing the minimum standards. This forces a certain standard to be maintained.

Which exercise to do, depends on age, physical fitness, availability of facilities, and many other factors. Problems, like arthritis, also impose limitations. For older people, we recommend low impact exercise, to put less stress on joints, and to prevent osteoarthritis. Swimming and cycling are probably two of the best low impact exercises.

My advice for managing your exercise program, and ensuring at least moderate success, is as follows:

Most of us hate to exercise alone, so find a partner or a group. It makes things more interesting and gives incentive to show up. In my practice, I contract out the exercise to some hot, female exercise instructors, as incentive for at least my male patients. It works! My other patients find exercise groups to join, in their favourite activity. This could be golf, cycling, scuba diving, tennis, or just hiking.

Make it regular. This is harder than it sounds, especially with more people involved. Logistics is always a problem. It's best to have one or two dedicated days so that people don't forget and schedule other things. There must be some commitment from all those involved.

Pick an exercise you enjoy. If you find it a chore, you will give it up shortly. What if you don't like anything? This is sometimes a problem for some sedentary people. I suggest pairing it with something you like. One girl, who worked for the CIA, had trouble incentivising her rather overweight boyfriend to exercise, so she made sure that before each workout, she would have a very vigorous workout in bed first. Very soon, the boyfriend was looking forward to each session, and would never cancel on her. Besides, there was a double benefit, because they each burned 200 Kcal before the exercise session even started!

Another essential is not to pair group exercise programs with eating and drinking binges after the event. There is a local golf course that has a 19th hole where weary golfers can put back on all the calories they lost, and more! After cycling for hours, it would be such a waste to end with beer drinking. At 43 Kcal per 100 gm in alcohol, it would not be difficult to put all the lost calories back on with a few pints. I suggest to end with no more than one beer, and after that, switch to ice tea with lemon, without sugar.

Variety is also the key to regularity. Cycle with different people, or take different routes, or cycle in different countries. Make it interesting! I am constantly looking for new cycling friends. I also take the opportunity to cycle whenever I am overseas for any reason. Recently, I explored the East German countryside around Fulda, and also cycled all around Vienna.

Invest in some equipment. This is also an incentive to pursue an activity so as not to let the equipment go to waste. This does not always work though. I have a rich Indonesian friend that bought a really expensive bicycle, rode it twice, and then never found the time to cycle again. On the other hand, I have 5 bicycles, and they never pass a week without getting used.

Time must be created. Don't tell yourself, "I will exercise when I have a break in my busy schedule," or, "I will exercise when I am less busy." You will never find time to be less busy, or have a break in your schedule. You must create it and prioritize it. Otherwise, forget it, and just resign yourself to getting fat and flabby, and suffering the consequences. Remember, "You reap what you sow."

In Summary:

- Diabetes can occasionally be cured by lifestyle changes alone.
- It demands strict discipline, in both diet and exercise.
- It has to be constantly maintained; otherwise, diabetes will relapse.
- Most people can't keep it up.
- There are easier ways to manage the disease.
- Lifestyle changes to lower blood sugar is a means of control and not a cure. If you don't maintain it, your diabetes will come back with a vengeance.
- It's possible to go down this route if you are merely pre-diabetic or your diabetes is very mild.

Chapter 6

Is Medicine the Solution?

In 1922, Banting and Best discovered insulin and started using it to treat diabetes. This development saved many lives. Before this, diabetes was a death sentence for many patients. Unless the diabetes was mild enough to be controlled solely by strict diet, complications soon followed, and death came swiftly.

Insulin was the very first weapon doctors had, but this was soon followed by the discovery of oral hypoglycemic medications, like biguanides and sulphonylureas, which could control the mild and moderate forms of the disease, and avoid the pain and inconvenience of frequent insulin injections.

Patients like it. Oral medications are painless and convenient. Most times, you take it once a day, and perhaps twice. It's an easy regime, and patients are lulled into a false sense of security. Meanwhile, the clock ticks down on a veritable time bomb.

Medications all have side effects. They don't really protect against vascular and other complications, and in 50% of cases, you will deteriorate and end up being on insulin. These are proven statistics. The first line drug is metformin. It is an excellent drug and is inexpensive. Side effects are rare, though lactic acidosis can happen rarely. If you are a type 2 diabetic, of normal weight or slim, and well controlled on metformin only, then you probably should just stick to that. It will reduce your HbA1c by about 1.5%.

It's another story if you are obese. Obesity adds on a whole other set of risks, and even mild diabetes can multiply your risks. If you are overweight or obese, and a mild diabetic, then losing the weight might just turn your diabetes around. If you are terribly disciplined, then diet and exercise might work, but most people are not that disciplined and cannot sustain a strict lifestyle on their own.

The surgical option is a good one for the obese, mild to moderate diabetic, as it makes keeping to a sustainable diet much easier, leads to rapid weight loss, and will, in the vast majority of cases, reverse the diabetes.

Sulphonylureas are also an old class of drugs, which are cheap and popular. They were the first widely used oral diabetic drugs. They stimulate the pancreatic islet cells to produce more insulin. In some patients, the insulin production is a problem, but I have measured the endogenous insulin production in every patient, using a test called the C peptide. Most patients are actually producing lots of insulin, and the main problem is insulin resistance. Another problem with sulphonylureas is that they can cause hypoglycemia, which can be a nuisance. I also wonder about the long-term effects of constant stimulation of the islet cells. It's like whipping a tired horse. The islet cells may just burn out over time, and production of insulin would decrease and be more resistant to stimulation. Other troublesome side effects include weight gain, and interaction with a host of other drugs. What's more, there is no conclusive evidence that the drug protects against cardiovascular complications of diabetes.

Discovery of the role of GLP-1, and the role it plays to decrease blood sugar and increase insulin production, have given us two new classes of drugs. The first are the GLP-1 agonists. One example is Victoza. The body produces its own GLP-1, and these drugs are similar to it, and act on the same receptors. GLP-1, however, is a peptide or string of amino acids, and if you take it orally, it just gets digested. So, GLP-agonists have to be injected, and this is not that popular with patients

Is Medicine the Solution?

because you might as well be on insulin, and the drug is also expensive.

On the positive side, the drug can result in moderate weight loss. The downside is that nausea and vomiting can be a troublesome side effect. Realistically, very few patients would be keen on an injectable that caused nausea. This is despite the fact that this is one of the few drugs that does lower cardiovascular risks.

A more convenient development are the DPP-4 inhibitors (dipeptidyl peptidase 4 inhibitors). Their effect is to increase incretin levels like GLP-1 and GIP. They do this by stopping the breakdown of these hormones.

On the whole, this is a good class of drugs and is reasonably effective in bringing down blood sugars. There are side effects, of course. Adverse effects include nasopharyngitis, headache, nausea, heart failure, hypersensitivity, and skin reactions. There is also a 58% increased risk of developing acute pancreatitis, and some worry about increased risk of pancreatic cancer, although this has only been seen in animals.

These drugs are often prescribed in a convenient combination pill, with various doses of metformin added into the pill, so that the patient only has to take one tablet rather than several.

They have some advantages to the GLP agonists because they can be taken orally. However, their effect is mild, and only reduce by 0.7 to 0.8%. Side effects are headaches and increased risk of infection, and it has no weight lowering effect. The effect on cardiovascular risks of diabetes are unknown. Most likely, there is no effect.

The latest class of drugs are the gliflozins, which are SGLT-2 inhibitors. SGLT-1 and SGLT-2 are proteins that cause reabsorption of glucose in the kidneys; so if you block them, sugar is passed into the urine rather than being reabsorbed into the blood stream. SGLT-1 is responsible for 10% of the reabsorption, while SGLT-2 does 90% of the job, so it makes sense to block SGLT-2.

Passing all that sugar into the urine does have some downsides, and side effects are mycotic infections of the genitals, urinary tract infections, and osmotic diuresis, which means that you are going to pee a lot and frequently.

More critically, the FDA issued a 2015 warning about increased risk of diabetic ketoacidosis (DKA). This is because reducing circulating glucose reduces endogenous insulin secretion. It can also cause euglycemic DKA, through renal tubular absorption of ketone bodies. One of the drugs, called canagliflozin, also causes decreased mineral bone density, which can increase risk of fractures.

Compared to sulphonylureas and insulin, this class of drugs does lower the risk of hypoglycemia.

On the positive side, it can lower the risk of amputation, and it does lower cardiovascular risk by about 20%. This does not match the 50% drop in cardiovascular risk achieved by metabolic surgery. This is one of the better drugs, but still, like all drugs, there are problems with it. I would like to mention two other classes of drugs, which are far less popular today, though they had their day in the sun in the past.

Thiazolidinediones (TZD) are also called glitazones. They act by a complex mechanism to influence insulin sensitive genes. In short, they improve the utilization of glucose by the cells. They are quite powerful and can reduce HbA1C by 1.5 to 2.0%. An example of this class of drugs is rosiglitazone (Avandia).

The problem is the safety issue. The greatest concern is the increase in the number of severe cardiac events in patients on this drug. This led to a 2010 suspension by the EU.

Is Medicine the Solution?

Another member of this class, troglitazone, was withdrawn in 1990, because it caused hepatitis and liver damage.

The saga of this drug demonstrates several points. Firstly, although the idea of a magic pill is very appealing, drugs are always a two-edged sword. My own philosophy is that one should make do with as little medication as possible. They all have the propensity to harm you, as they do not have a direct effect on insulin.

The last class of drugs I want to discuss are the alpha glucosidase inhibitors. They are not strictly hypoglycemic agents, as they do not have a direct effect on the secretion or sensitivity of insulin. They slow the absorption of starch in the small intestines so that glucose from starch breakdown enters the blood stream more slowly, and the impaired insulin response of the diabetic has more time to cope with the sugar influx.

These drugs are only of use in early and mild diabetes. They have a very mild effect on the HbA1C, and reduce it by 0.5% to 1% at best. An example of this class of drugs is acarbose.

These medications are rarely prescribed in the USA, as they cause bloating and flatulence, which many patients find intolerable. They are more popular in Europe. They do have a mild weight loss effect.

At this point, let us summarize the pros and cons of using medication.

Advantages of medical treatment of diabetes:

- Easy and convenient, as long as you don't get on insulin
- Cheap in the short term
- Not scary
- Perceived to be safe
- Easily available
- Costs covered by some countries

Downside of medical treatment:

- Lose 10 years of your life
- May not protect against cardiovascular complications
- Doubles cancer risk
- Controls but doesn't cure
- 50% eventually requiring insulin injections
- Cannot reverse complications of diabetes
- Expensive in the long run, especially when you calculate the lifelong costs and costs of treatment of the complications of diabetes
- Has side effects
- Becomes an incurable disease (diabetes) when you take the medical route

Juggling these drugs, and trying to optimize them for individual diabetics, is the obsession of the endocrinologist. They have made it into a complex science, which only they understand. In medicine, when the treatment of a disease becomes complicated with endless options and endless variations, this usually means that the solution isn't down this route. We need to make a quantum jump and get to the destination of remission or cure, and the answer does not lie in a pill or combination of pills.

So now we have to examine the worst-case scenario. What happens when your diabetes gets worse, and you cannot control your blood sugars on oral medication? The conventional solution is insulin injections. Let's take a look at what that is like. We shall discuss this in the next chapter.

Chapter 7

Insulin: The Curse of the Needles

Insulin was life-saving. Before insulin, everyone with diabetes died. It was as fatal as heart disease or cancer. The introduction of insulin was a game changer and made it possible for diabetics to stay alive. Before the 1920s, everyone with diabetes died, because there were no good treatments.

Insulin was first used for the treatment of diabetes in Toronto, Canada, by Sir Frederick G. Banting and Charles H. Best, and was subsequently purified by James B. Collip. Banting was actually an orthopedic surgeon. He discovered insulin in 1921. Insulin was first used on patients on January 11, 1922. In 1923, Banting received the Nobel Prize, at the age of 32. He was the youngest laureate in the field of physiology/medicine. Insulin was commercially available in the USA by 1923.

Longer acting insulins became available soon after; in 1983, it became lab synthesized and didn't need to be extracted from pigs or cows.

Oral hypoglycemic drugs soon became available, starting with tolbutamide, which was marketed in 1950, in Germany; and Metformin, in 1959, though it was not approved in the USA until the 1990s.

Although the history is pretty interesting, I think that what you want to know is what it is like using insulin, and whether it is a way of life that you can live with. So I will skip the history lesson and come back to the here and now.

All type 1 diabetics need insulin. Fifty percent of type 2 diabetics would slowly deteriorate and would eventually require insulin. This statistic would bring a broad smile to the pharmaceutical industry and the average diabetes doctor who does no surgery. It is a hugely profitable business for them. Many diabetic specialists would actually like you to go on insulin sooner than later, because then you become dependent on them; and most general practitioners would rather not manage insulin therapy as it is time consuming and risky for them. It is estimated that 100 million people worldwide are on insulin.

For the patient, however, a life on insulin injections is far from rosy. First of all, pricking yourself with an insulin syringe is not the only pain you have to endure. You are advised never to give yourself insulin unless you know your blood sugar level. This is to avoid over dosing or under dosing yourself, which could have disastrous consequences. You will thus be tied to a bag of insulin equipment, which would include vials, syringes, needles, insulin pens, swabs, test strips, lancets, and your glucometer. You have to have access to your life support system all day. Your whole life will be tied to checking sugar levels, calculating dosage, and injecting yourself. It's far from a relaxed lifestyle.

It is actually difficult to have a regular regime, because everything you do or don't do can affect your blood sugar level. This includes activity, exercise, timing of food and drinks, type of food, quantity of food, stress, hormones, etc. The regulation of blood sugar is extremely complex. Imagine the problems you will have when you are travelling. What will you do if you lose your insulin bag?

Yes, you might actually die if you did not get your insulin. Type 1s will not survive more than 7 to 10 days or so, and will die an awful death. Type 2s might last longer, depending on how bad they are.

Insulin: The Curse of the Needles

For type 2 diabetics, the milder ones might get away with one long-acting insulin dose a day, and supplement that with an oral hypoglycemic. The more serious diabetics will need to supplement this 2 or 3 times a day, with short-acting insulin at every meal, and will also need to check their blood sugar before each injection. That adds up to a lot of pricks!

Let's take an average patient on one dose of long-acting insulin and a top-up every meal. That's 1,460 injections per year, and the same number of finger pricks. That's nearly 44,000 injections and 44,000 finger pricks, if you are lucky enough to live 30 years!

Wouldn't you want to avoid all that pain if you could?

Insulin can be given from a vial, with a syringe and needle, or more conveniently, it comes in a pen, which is easier to manage. However, the pen is 30% more expensive, and insulin therapy is already very costly.

So, who gets to go on insulin? If you are on two oral medications, and your HbA1C is more than 7% after 2 or 3 months, your doctor would likely suggest insulin. If your HbA1C is more than 10%, he would probably start you at once.

Let's now talk about some of the complications of being on insulin. Being on insulin is a balancing act. If you give too little, your blood sugar is high and you feel bad. If it keeps being high, there are long-term consequences. If you give too much, you get hypoglycemia. You will feel weak, faint, and irritable, and if it really gets too low, you may even pass out. If it gets really low, you might die.

Insulin makes you hungry, and you eat more and may gain weight. You feel weak, so you exercise less as well. You may also get headaches and skin problems. You may suffer from an insulin allergy and insulin edema.

If you are not totally aseptic in your injection technique, you may get infections at the injection sites. This may progress to an abscess, which needs surgical drainage. If you inject into the same spot too many times, you may be hardening the fat in that area, producing a lump or a depression. This is called lipodystrophy. If you keep injecting into an area of hardened fat, your insulin effect may be decreased because the absorption is slowed down.

It's pretty common to get complications when you inject yourself 1,460 times a year. Don't forget all the painful finger pricks.

The worst downside of being on insulin is the increased cancer risk. Seven common cancers are involved.

High insulin levels increase the risk of colorectal cancer, which is the number 1 cancer in men, and number 2 in women. Precancerous growths, called adenomas or polyps, are increased by 17% to 42% on colonoscopy.

Gastric or stomach cancer is increased by 69% to 101%, depending on how high the insulin levels are.

There is a 2 to 3-fold increased risk for breast cancer. There is a similar risk for endometrial cancer, and 10-fold increase in early premalignant changes in endometrial cells. There is a 45-fold increase in type 1 endometrial cancer. There is also an increased risk of ovarian cancer. Women on insulin should really think about getting off this hormone. For men, prostate cancer becomes a major risk. With low levels of insulin, there is a 2.55-fold increase, and a 5.62-fold increase in those with the highest levels.

If you have been infected with the hepatitis B virus, and if your insulin level is high, you have a 2.4-fold increased risk of liver cancer.

The increased risk is quite significant and also applies to type 2 diabetics with high insulin resistance, who also have high insulin levels in their blood.

Finally, let's talk about costs. So many people in the USA can't afford to pay for insulin. The cost of being on insulin now averages about 400 US dollars per month. The price has doubled in the last 5 years. Insulin pens cost 30% more than insulin vials. Interestingly, some type 2 diabetics may need more insulin than those with type 1, because of very high insulin resistance.

If you calculate for one year, it is $4800 and for 30 years it is $144,000. This doesn't even begin to address the cost of treating complications. Reversing or curing your diabetes, and coming off insulin, would be a real bargain. Cost savings would be tremendous.

Why is the cost of insulin so high?

There is a monopoly. Only 3 companies dominate 90% of the world market—Eli Lilly, Novo Nordisk, and Sanofi. Only China and India were able to have their own domestic production.

There are no generic insulins. Creating biosimilar molecules are complicated and more expensive. After all, it is just a polypeptide.

The big 3 use pay-for-delay schemes and lawsuits to keep others out of the market.

The big 3 file very many patents to combat patent expiry. For instance, Sanofi has filed 74 patent applications for Lantus alone—so they have a competition-free monopoly for 37 years! Patents usually expire in 20 years.

Politics. The drug companies spend millions on lobbying politicians. This allows them to practice price gouging without political interference.

Price fixing. They all agree to keep prices high.

They bribe the physicians to influence their practices. These are disguised as loyalty rewards, research grants, sponsorship for conferences and educational activities, etc.

Payment for influence or silence. Opinion leaders, influencers, and patient advocacy organizations take pharma cash. The American Diabetic Association, for instance, has accepted huge amounts of cash from pharma. This makes them keep quiet about the less than ethical behavior of these companies, and also to keep silent about new, game-changing innovation, like surgery to reverse diabetes. Despite the strong pharma lobby, the ADA has come up with a strong statement supporting metabolic surgery to reverse or cure diabetes. The only problem is that this document has not been circulated to the end user—the patient.

To fight this situation is not easy. Pharma has a lot of money and will fight tooth and nail to protect their interests. We will discuss the politics and economics of this in another chapter.

I think the best that a diabetic patient can do is to look after his/her own interests. Fix your diabetes. Get off drugs and insulin so that you are not dependent on pharmaceuticals. After metabolic surgery, all you need is a healthy lifestyle.

Why enrich the pharmaceutical industry at your expense?

Chapter 8

How Does Surgery Reverse Diabetes?

The fact that metabolic surgery has a dramatic effect on blood sugar levels cannot be contested. The effect of metabolic surgery kicks in immediately. A dramatic effect is seen the day after the operation, and it gets even better the second and third days. Most patients achieve normal or near normal blood sugar readings the second or third day when they get out of hospital. Most times, patients will not even require oral medication at discharge.

Is it due to starvation or weight loss?

Several studies, done largely by non-surgeons, have tried to explain away the dramatic results of surgery by claiming that the same effects can be produced by starvation and weight loss. There is some evidence for the former but none whatsoever for the latter. Let's first deal with the idea that starvation is the mechanism of diabetes reversal.

It is true that if a diabetic goes on a dramatic starvation regime, his blood sugar will drop. After all, diabetes is a disease of sugar metabolism, and the main problem is the body's inability to process sugar. If there is no food going down, then there is no sugar to process, and the blood sugar will be low. Think about it. This is not a sustainable situation. You can't cure diabetes by starving. Surgery does not correct the diabetes by starving the patient. When the patient resumes liquids, or even progresses to soft solids, the blood sugar stays down and may even go lower. If the effect of the surgery was really due only to starvation, then the blood sugars would rise as soon as the patient gets back on food of any kind, whether solid or liquid. There would be no possibility of maintaining blood sugars after resumption of normal diet. The truth is that the reverse happens. The patient, after surgery, is able to maintain normal blood sugars, even after resumption of liquids and, subsequently, a solid diet. This is, therefore, just another attempt by non-surgeons to distort the facts and mislead the poor diabetic. They are trying to say that the same effect can be achieved just by not eating. Firstly, this is impossible as a means to control diabetes, as it is unsustainable; and secondly, it is just not true.

Next, we shall deal with the theory that the reversal of diabetes after surgery is due to weight loss. The dramatic time frame of the changes flies against this theory as well. Patients, after metabolic surgery, see a dramatic reduction in blood sugar levels almost immediately, often in days. How much can a post-operative patient lose in 3 days? Perhaps one or two kilograms at most. Recently, I did see one patient lose 6 kg in a week, after a sleeve resection, but that is rare indeed.

As every doctor and even every diabetic patient knows, losing one or 2 kilograms isn't going to make a dramatic impact on the blood sugar levels; yet most patients see a dramatic drop in fasting sugar, to normal or near normal, within days.

Once again, we must come to the conclusion that greater events are afoot than the simplistic idea that the reversal of diabetes is due to weight loss. The analysis of the effectiveness of various bariatric procedures, in regard to the reversal of diabetes, also sheds some light on the effect of weight loss on diabetes. Procedures such as gastric balloon and gastric band will lead to weight loss, and have some effect on diabetes for sure. The rate of reversal, however, is far lower than those achieved by the more metabolically active operations.

Generally, procedures that do not lead to changes in gut hormones, are far less effective. One evidence of this is that a gastric band has resolution rates of less than 50%, and a sleeve gastrectomy leads to total remission in about 65% to 70% of patients. A gastric bypass, which has a much stronger metabolic effect, can reverse diabetes in the overweight or obese diabetic, in about 95% of patients. The most drastic procedures of all—the duodenal switch or the biliopancreatic bypass—would almost guarantee a reversal. Ninety-nine percent or more would be reversed.

These figures tell one thing: Some change in hormonal balance is required to reverse the sugar balance in the body. We need to recalibrate the balance of hormones that regulate sugar. It's not just a question of weight loss. On the other hand, weight loss does reduce all the factors that cause insulin resistance, and will lock in the gains that accrue from the surgery. Getting back to normal weight really never hurt anyone. For diabetics, it can only make the sugar situation better.

Hormonal Changes Brought About by Metabolic Surgery

We talked about gut hormones in the previous chapter. These hormones are super important in regulating blood sugar, and we can tweak these hormones when we do metabolic surgery.

How does metabolic surgery change the gut hormones? First, we must understand in which direction we want to change these hormones. The aim is to eliminate the hormones that raise blood sugar, and enhance the hormones that reduce blood sugar.

The hormones that raise blood sugar after a meal are in the foregut. This is the region of the gut that first meets the food we take. It consists of the stomach and the duodenum, which is the first part of the small intestine. The first target for intervention is the ghrelin receptor in the fundus of the stomach. The fundus is a pouch at the upper part of the stomach, next to the spleen. In the sleeve gastrectomy, this part of the stomach is removed. In the bypass, it is excluded from the food stream. Either way, the secretion of ghrelin, which is a hunger hormone, can be reduced or eliminated.

The second hormonal mechanism is the duodenum. The duodenum and the proximal small bowel have receptors that produce hormones, which increase blood sugar after a meal. When food passes through these areas of the gut, hormones—called anti-incretins—are produced, which then raise the blood sugar level. Scientists are not entirely sure which hormones are responsible, or how many, but glucagon, which is produced by the alpha cells in the pancreas, is probably one of them. Other hormones implicated are cholecystokinin and secretin. This is the basis of the *foregut mechanism* of blood sugar control. When operations like the Roux-en-Y bypass, gastric mini bypass, or duodenal switch are performed, food is diverted so that it doesn't pass through these areas of the gut. The post-prandial rise in blood sugar is thus eliminated. This is one of the really powerful mechanisms underlying the control of blood sugar levels after a gastric bypass.

Interestingly, this mechanism is left intact after a sleeve resection; yet a strong blood sugar lowering effect is seen immediately after a sleeve resection. This shows that much remains unknown about metabolic surgery. We also haven't figured out the mechanism of the remarkable blood pressure lowering effects, and cholesterol lowering effects, of metabolic surgery.

The other powerful mechanism underlying the remarkable blood sugar lowering effects of metabolic surgery is the so-called *hind gut mechanism*. The lower part of the ileum, or terminal ileum in medical jargon, has a bunch of receptors, which control the production incretins. These are hormones that have a blood sugar lowering effect. It does this by various mechanisms. These hormones are also enhanced after the performance of metabolic surgery.

How Does Surgery Reverse Diabetes?

The most important of these hormones is GLP-1, or glucagon-like polypeptide 1. This hormone is secreted by the lower small bowel, and has the effect of lowering blood sugar, increasing insulin secretion, decreasing insulin resistance, and protecting the insulin secreting beta cells of the pancreas. In short, it has a strong antidiabetic effect. The pharma industry has already exploited this in the development of two classes of drugs. One class is the GLP-1 agonists, or drugs that behave like GLP-1. The drug, Victoza, or liraglutide, is such a drug. It has several disadvantages. Firstly, it has to be injected; and secondly, it causes nausea. Natural GLP-1 does not cause any nausea, and it is enhanced by metabolic surgery. It is produced by the L cells of the small intestine. Other incretins that are likely to have a role in reversing diabetes are GIP, which is gastric inhibitory polypeptide, or glucose-dependent insulinotropic polypeptide. This hormone also has an incretin effect, but it may not work so well on type 2 diabetics. The other important hormone is PYY, or polypeptide YY. This hormone decreases appetite and slows gastric emptying, so it has a potent weight reduction effect, which of course helps in stabilizing the blood sugar. This hormone would exert an anti-diabetic effect over the longer term, rather than be responsible for the immediate drop in blood sugar seen after surgery.

Adiponectin is a hormone produced in fat cells. It has a role in energy metabolism and insulin production. All studies show that adiponectin is increased after weight loss, whether it is medical or surgical. This is a secondary effect. The hormone increases once you lose weight, and is not the result of the surgery per se.

It is clear that there are many other hormonal mechanisms involved, and we will very quickly find out what these are, considering the pace of research going on at present. This is probably one of the hottest areas being investigated in gastrointestinal physiology.

Effect of Surgery on Bile Acids

There are two other blood sugar lowering mechanisms. One of them is the increase in bile acid absorption after bypass surgery. This has an effect on lipid and carbohydrate metabolism. Increased bile acids in the circulation can halve the cholesterol levels, and also lead to increased insulin sensitivity. These effects usually kick in one to two weeks after surgery, and are not responsible for the early changes in blood glucose. Free bile acids are also increased in the terminal ileum, and this has an effect to increase GLP-1, which as mentioned before, is an incretin, and lowers blood sugar and increases insulin production. One of the reasons bile acid is increased in both the blood and the lower small bowel, is because there is less time for the bile to mix with the food. This leads to more bile acid absorption into the blood stream, and more of it leftover in the lower intestine.

Bacterial Changes in the Gut

Another effect is the change in the bacteria of the gut after metabolic surgery. This phenomenon may also be related to the increased bile acids in the bowel. A bacteria, called proteobacteria, is increased after bariatric surgery. This phenomenon is not seen after medical weight loss. This bacterial overgrowth somehow leads to an increased serum bile acid level, which has an incretin effect.

We realise that the mechanisms underlying the overall blood sugar lowering effect, after metabolic surgery, is complex, and that the last word has not been said. It involves not only weight loss but hormonal, bile, and bacterial effects, which all interact together to produce the remarkable reversal of diabetes. Although we do not yet fully understand everything about how it all works, we are all in agreement that it works!

There are many more interesting findings coming out about the issue of gut bacteria. Gut bacteria has a role in diabetes, but it also has a big role in obesity as well. In one classic experiment on twin rats, it was found that when the fatter rat fed on the stool of the thinner rat, he lost weight and became slim. The reverse also occurred. If the thin rat ate the stool of the fatter rat, he became fat. We can therefore conclude that the type of microbiological flora in the gut has something to do with weight maintenance, and not only maintenance of sugar levels. Actually, 3 types of bacteria have been identified, which may promote weight loss. They are Lactobacillus gasseri, Lactobacillus rhamnosus, and Bifidobacterium lactis. They are quite commonly found in commercial probiotic combinations. I do not think the effect on weight will be spectacular, but these bacteria may be useful for small scale weight loss or maintenance after bariatric and metabolic surgery.

This field is still being actively researched, and new findings are emerging all the time. We understand some of the mechanisms but not all of them. What cannot be disputed is that metabolic surgery is spectacularly successful, and that the results are objective, repeatable, and verifiable. There is no subjective element, because blood sugar, HbA1C, blood pressure, and cholesterol levels are measurable and objective end points.

Long-term studies again verify the cardiovascular protection, decreased cancer incidence, and increased longevity. These are all statistically proven, and are published in peer reviewed mainstream medical and scientific journals.

The medical community may not like it, but they will have a hard time refuting it, as they can't do any real studies showing the opposite.

Randomized Controlled Trials and Other Scientific Evidence

The RCT, or randomized controlled trial, is the highest form of scientific evidence, which verifies the efficacy of a medical or surgical treatment. More than twenty RCTs have been published comparing surgery to medical treatment. Most of these trials compare the results of bariatric or metabolic treatment to optimal medical treatment plus lifestyle changes. Without lifestyle changes, medical treatment would get a zero remission rate.

The results of all these trials prove conclusively that surgery is superior in every single study. These trials are not done by small obscure centres, or published in obscure journals. The best trials are all done by top institutions, and are published in the top journals, such as the New England Journal of Medicine, which is regarded as the very top medical journal, along with the Lancet.

This is not a textbook for medical professionals, and it is not aimed at doctors and those suffering from the disease, so I will not include tedious quotes or references from these studies.

We live in the internet age, and all scientific studies are available on Google, Internet Explorer, or other search engines.

Key words to use are: metabolic surgery for type 2 diabetes; randomized controlled trials; diabetes surgery; Philip Schauer, Stampede trial, Cleveland Clinic; Mingrone Italian Trial 2012; New England Medical Journal; etc.

If you are truly a person who wants to know the details, you can find it all on the internet.

The Stampede trial published 1-year, 3-year, and 5-year results, in the New England Medical Journal.

In 2016, the American Diabetic Association published a consensus statement on metabolic surgery in diabetes care. It was supported by 45 medical and surgical societies worldwide. Metabolic surgery was clearly supported in this statement as an equivalent to medical treatment or better, and should not be a last resort but an equivalent treatment, depending on the patient's choice. Actually, all studies show that the earlier the intervention, the better the results.

Finally, the greatest diabetes authority in the world can no longer ignore the evidence, and has endorsed it as probably the best treatment for diabetes we have at present.

Chapter 9

What Procedures Can Reverse or Cure Diabetes?

There are now a myriad of procedures that can reverse diabetes, and the list is ever growing. Older operations are also being constantly refined and made safer and more effective. Let's go through some of them. Almost all operations are done by keyhole or laparoscopic surgery nowadays. Some of them can be done by mini-laparoscopic surgery, which is also called needlescopic or pin-hole surgery.

Sleeve Gastrectomy

This is also known as vertical stapled gastrectomy. It was invented by my old friend, Michel Gagner, from Montreal, around 1997. This procedure was part of a larger procedure called duodenal switch. It was discovered serendipitously when Michel was unable to complete a duodenal switch on a difficult obese patient, and decided to stage the procedure, leaving the operation partly completed, having done the stomach resection but not the bypass part. The patient had a very good result despite not having the full operation. Since then, it has evolved and become a widely used, popular, and very safe stand-alone operation.

This is the simplest metabolic surgery procedure, and it has the lowest complication rate. The surgeon simply applies a row of titanium staples, parallel to the lesser curve of the stomach. The whole procedure takes about an hour or less.

I trained with Michel's team in Doha, and we were doing up to 8 sleeve operations a day, running two operating rooms. An analysis of more than a thousand cases showed complete resolution of diabetes in 65%, and partial remission in 30%. Only 5% of cases remained unchanged. That was in an unselected group, and patients were doing the operation mainly for obesity rather than diabetes. If proper case selection were done, the success rate would be far higher.

This operation is really good for reversal of mild to moderate diabetes, but it is not as good for reversing really severe diabetes.

The biggest advantage is that it is quick, not technically difficult, and it is reproducible and safe. The weight loss is about 40% of excess body weight on the average, and it is pretty good at reversing hypertension and high cholesterol, as well as diabetes.

It is now probably the most commonly done bariatric procedure in the world. If Michel Gagner could hold a patent on this procedure, he would be an oligarch today.

Gastric Bypass

There are many types of gastric bypass operations. These operations are more complicated than a sleeve resection, and take more time. They are also technically more difficult to perform, and they require a higher level of surgical training. The reason for this is that they all require the construction of one or more anastomosis. The anastomosis is the junction between one piece of gut and another. Most often, this is a junction between the stomach and the small bowel, or between one level of small bowel and another. In laymen terms, it can be considered the construction of a road junction.

Historically, the first successful gastric bypass for obesity was the Roux-en-Y gastric bypass. Cesar Roux, a Swiss surgeon, invented the Roux-en-Y in 1892, to treat obstruction. In the 1960s, Dr. Edward

What Procedures Can Reverse or Cure Diabetes?

Mason and Dr. Chikashi Ito noticed that patients lost weight after the operation. The first bariatric Roux-en-Y was done in 1967 by this pair. At that time, the operation was done by open surgery, with all the attendant technical difficulties, slow recovery, and post-operative pain. In 1985, there was a major revolution in the surgical world, with the advent of laparoscopic cholecystectomy, which revolutionized how surgery was performed. Most operations can now be done through tiny holes, with the operating view captured by tiny microchip cameras, and projected onto large, high definition screens. This was a quantum leap and a game changer in the field. We were fortunate to be in the forefront of this development.

Gastric bypass could not yet be done by laparoscopic surgery, till one historic moment in February 1992, when my team and I, at the National University of Singapore, performed the world's first laparoscopic totally intra-abdominal Billroth II gastrectomy. This event revolutionized stomach surgery, and made laparoscopic bariatric and metabolic surgery possible. Elements of the operation, such as the construction of the anastomosis between stomach and small bowel, underpin the development of the various gastric bypass operations done today.

This operation was presented to the surgical world in April of 1992, to a packed audience at the meeting of the SAGES (Society of American Gastrointestinal Endoscopic Surgeons), in Washington DC, and was published in September of the same year.

The principle of the gastric bypass is:

- To create a smaller stomach pouch.
- To join that pouch to the small bowel, distally bypassing a variable length of small intestine.

In this way, there is a restrictive and a malabsorptive element introduced to promote weight loss. Concurrently, it produces a very strong antidiabetic effect by altering the gut hormones. These effects are produced because the food stream is diverted. To put it simply, the food that used to trigger gut hormones that raise blood sugar, no longer pass the receptors that trigger them. They are diverted to parts of the bowel that have receptors for incretins or antidiabetic hormones, which have the opposite effect of bringing down blood sugar instead. The effect is powerful and dramatic.

The various bypass procedures thus trigger both the foregut and the hindgut mechanisms to reverse diabetes, making them very powerful anti-diabetic procedures. This contrasts with the sleeve operations, where the food still passes through the duodenum and triggers the anti-incretins, which raise blood sugar.

The antidiabetic effect of a bypass operation is thus more powerful, and we use it for the more severe diabetic. It also seems to work better for the lower BMI patient, where the aim is to reverse the diabetes rather than to cause massive weight loss.

The three types of bypasses commonly used will be discussed below. Roux-en-Y bypass – This is the laparoscopic version of the original, highly successful, open surgery equivalent, done since the 1960s. It is a well proven technique, but it is technically probably the more difficult to perform of the common bariatric procedures. Nevertheless, it is in most bariatric surgeons' repertoires. The stomach pouch is made very small, with about 50 to 100cc capacity. A distal loop of jejunum is truncated and pulled up to join to the stomach pouch. The proximal loop of small bowel is then joined much lower down, to allow the biliopancreatic juices to rejoin the food stream distally. I know this is quite a difficult concept to understand if you are not a surgeon. I therefore will not elaborate further, because these technical details are as useful to the consumer as the algorithms inside an iPhone. There are two anastomosis; so, technically, there is twice the chance of an anastomotic problem, and the configuration of the change creates two potential mesenteric defects that potentially can cause hernias, and most surgeons close these defects. The operation, therefore, is quite involved and would take longer to perform.

Mini gastric bypass – This is also known as the single anastomosis bypass. This is a simplification of the Roux-en-Y, and was not accepted for a long time, but it has now proven itself and joined the mainstream. Dr. Robert Rutledge, of Las Vegas, was the pioneer of this operation and has been its main advocate worldwide. I started doing this operation as early as 1997, but he was the original pioneer. There are many variations of this operation, but in principle, the small bowel is not truncated, and just brought up as a loop and anastomosed to a new stomach pouch, created by staples. The new stomach pouch is longer and elongated, and the anastomosis is done lower down, which makes it easier. The single anastomosis reduces the problems from having two anastomosis, but if leaks occur at this site, they can be more problematic to manage. This operation also doesn't create any mesenteric defects as potential hernia sites. Generally, it takes about 30 minutes to an hour longer to do than the gastric sleeve. The configuration of the bypass is like that of the Billroth II gastrectomy.

Duodenal jejunal bypass (DJ bypass) – Both of the previous operations leave a substantial part of the stomach behind, and out of reach of any endoscopic surveillance. This poses a problem in countries with high incidence of stomach cancer. In these countries, a DJ bypass is becoming popular, as the entire remaining stomach is accessible to a gastroscope. The operation starts with a sleeve gastrectomy. The bypass occurs distal to the pyloric sphincter and can be done either in a Roux-en-Y double anastomosis configuration or in a single anastomosis configuration (Billroth 2) This type of bypass is much less commonly done than the first two. Stomach cancer incidence has dropped drastically in most countries because of the practice of Helicobacter pylori eradication. This bacteria has been identified as the main cause of stomach cancer. Bypass operations have both a restrictive and a malabsorptive function. You can lose up to 70% of your excess body weight after a bypass. A 2007 study, in the New

England Journal of Medicine, shows a 40% reduction in death rate compared to those obese individuals who did not have a bypass. The effect on diabetes can be phenomenal with reversal, sometimes within one to two days.

Duodenal Switch and Biliopancreatic Bypass

These are pretty drastic surgical operations, meant originally for the super obese. They have a restrictive element like the bypass, in terms of a small gastric pouch but a more drastic small bowel diversion.

One feature of both operations is the creation of a very long biliopancreatic loop of small bowel, which food doesn't pass. The bile and pancreatic juices join the digestive stream, only 75cm to 150cm from the end of the ileum. This configuration causes a very strong check on digestion and absorption of food.

Both these operations lead to massive weight loss and have the strongest effect on diabetes of any procedure. The rate of reversal or cure of diabetes is from 98% to 100%, but it comes at a price. No, I am not talking about money. The effect on digestion and absorption of nutrients is pretty drastic.

These operations are, of course, more difficult to perform, and they have a higher complication rate.

Ileal Transposition

This is a very innovative procedure, developed by my old friend, Aureo Ludovico de Paula, from Brazil. The terminal part of the small bowel, or ileum, is resected and transposed more proximally. This transposed area of bowel contains the receptors that trigger the production of incretins such as GLP-1. These anti-diabetic hormones are thus triggered promptly after a meal, and bring down the blood sugar. It is usually done together with a sleeve resection, or at least resection of the fundus of the stomach to avoid the side effect of vomiting. This operation gained some traction in India but is still considered somewhat experimental.

There are two other procedures I would like to mention, which may have an effect on diabetes but are mainly done for weight loss. The anti-diabetic effects of these procedures are mild.

Gastric Banding

This was a very popular weight loss procedure for about 2 decades, but it has since fallen from favor. It is a purely restrictive procedure, consisting of putting a silicone inflatable band round the upper stomach. The band is adjustable by injecting more or less saline into it via a subcutaneous port. It was a reasonably successful operation for weight loss, though less effective than either the sleeve or bypass operations. As an anti-diabetic procedure, it is much less successful, as it does not produce the hormone changes required to really reverse the diabetes. Nevertheless, in 2004, one group in Georgia published that diabetes was reversed by 66% in one year, and 80% in two years. This may be due to the weight loss alone. What was interesting was that hypertension was reversed in 59%. All this was achieved with an average weight loss of 39.2%. What this study shows is that weight loss alone can have a drastic effect on diabetes.

Gastric Balloon

This is an inflatable silicone ball that can be installed in the stomach as a weight reduction device. Its main function is to slow gastric emptying and to occupy space in the stomach to produce a sensation of satiety. It is a weight loss device and not an anti-diabetic device.

New evidence shows that a gastric balloon can also reverse diabetes. A recent study presented in the SAGES meeting, in 2018, from the Chinese University of Hong Kong, shows a 35.7% remission rate for diabetes. Another study by a different group, published by the American Diabetic Association, also shows a significant reversal of hypertension.

For those who are totally averse to surgery, the gastric balloon is an option to consider. It is installed and removed through the mouth, like any endoscopic procedure, and takes only 10 to 15 minutes. Older balloons last about 6 months, but Spatz has a balloon that can last one year and is adjustable.

A recent US FDA comparative trial showed the Spatz adjustable balloon to produce more weight loss than all the rest. It can produce a spectacular 54% to 67% excess body weight loss, compared to 38% loss, using its nearest rival, the Oberon balloon. We have yet to receive reports on the Spatz balloon's effect on diabetes.

The problem with balloons is that weight can be regained after the balloon is removed, and thus the diabetes can recur. On the other hand, balloons can be done sequentially and multiple times.

Endo Barrier

This is a 60 cm Teflon sleeve, which is installed in the duodenal bulb and runs all the way down the jejunum. The main purpose is to cover the lining of the duodenum to produce the foregut mechanism of diabetic control, which you get from a gastric bypass. It can reduce the HbA1c by about 1.5%, which is not bad for an endoscopic, non-surgical option. The downside, of course, is that it is temporary and cannot be left in long term, and has to be removed.

New methods of reversing diabetes are being developed constantly, and this is a very dynamic field. The general trend is toward less invasive, safer, and quicker options. We must also be cognizant that the bigger surgical procedures give a bigger and more long-lasting anti-diabetic effect for now. We cannot predict what will be available in the future.

Take-Home Message

The diabetic patient really has a lot of choice as to procedures. It is best to navigate these options with an expert, although many patients have already made up their mind what procedure they want, even before they see their surgeon. The internet is full of information, and you can access it and read everything—but caveat emptor. Some of the stuff you read isn't exactly scientifically verified.

A metabolic or bariatric surgeon is the best person to run through the advantages and disadvantages of all the choices, and to help you pick the one that best suits your situation.

Chapter 10

The Conquest of Fear

There are generally 3 main reasons diabetic patients shun getting an instant surgical fix for their disease. The first is ignorance and disbelief. The second is the cost; and the third, which is the most difficult to overcome, is fear.

People have a primitive and almost instinctive psychological aversion to surgery. This has not been helped by the historical perspective of the evolution of surgery. In ancient times, surgery was largely feared and shunned because it was extremely painful—there was no anesthesia. It took a long time to recover after surgery, because it was done by the open technique. And the mortality and complication rate was very high.

People did not agree to surgery till the disease was life threatening and there was no choice. Sadly, this attitude has persisted till today, although science has now changed everything. Nowadays, it is often true that not having surgery would be much more injurious to health than doing surgery. In many cases, doing surgery early would cure previously incurable diseases, save lives, increase the life expectancy, and prevent future complications that would be far more deleterious to the patient than the surgery itself.

Let's examine some of the advances that have created the favorable situation that we have today.

The first massive advance we have is safe anesthesia. Surgery is very much less dreaded today because we have general anesthesia. We go to sleep, and when we wake up, the job is done, and you have literarily time travelled past the whole event.

In the early 19th century, surgery was still an excruciating experience. Patients had to be tied down or held down, and there was hardly anything to help the patient through the terrible pain of the experience—except maybe a bottle of whisky for the patient, a bottle for the surgeon, and a bullet to bite on. Four big guys were required to hold the patient down. Usually, more than half of the patients who went for surgery expired. Although this image still sticks in the primitive subconscious of people—and we all have a natural aversion to being cut up anyway—the reality is far different today.

The game changer actually happened a long time ago, on October 16, 1846, to be exact. A dentist named William Thomas Green Morton, put a patient, Edward Gilbert Abbott, to sleep using ether. The surgeon, Dr. John Collins Warren, then proceeded to remove a neck tumor from the patient. The event occurred in an operating room at the Massachusetts General Hospital in Boston, where I trained, and it was later renamed the Ether Dome. The room exists to this day, and is now used to conduct lectures on molecular genetics. When I was training there, I used to attend these lectures weekly.

The operation was a huge success, and word spread fast. That single event changed everything. It made surgery comfortable for the patient, as well as for the surgeon. The surgeon was no longer under time pressure, and could do a meticulous slow dissection with much better results and safety. The whole field of anesthesia developed after this.

Nowadays, anesthesia is super safe, and the patient really has little to worry about. Mortality is as low as 7 per million anesthetic episodes. I myself have undergone anesthesia four times; I don't remember a single bit of any of the operations, and I have had no side effects from the medication at all. Each time, it was a really anticlimactic experience. It was like taking a nap and waking up.

About 10 years ago, I donated a kidney to my brother. Even though I knew it was relatively safe, I was still afraid. Now I realize that it was just the primitive, historical, and cultural instincts acting up. I was put to sleep in the waiting room, and a moment later, I woke up in the same waiting room—I never even saw the operating room, and the operation was over. I felt a little pain when I woke up, which was great as it confirmed I was still alive!

Several years later, I went for a throat operation to relieve my sleep apnoea. This time, the anesthesia was even more amazing. I was put to sleep in my room before I even left for the operating suite, and I woke up back in my room. I don't even remember the journey to the OR and back. That's how amazing general anesthesia is today. The anxiety and fear can be totally removed, and surgery can be as anxiety free as going to a hairdresser or a spa. Anesthesia has now become an extremely refined science, and much of the dread of surgery can be totally eliminated.

The next fear, of course, is the pain of the post-operative period. The good news is that a revolution in surgery, starting in the mid-eighties in the last century, has changed the post-operative experience tremendously for the better. The revolution, nowadays, is called the *Laparoscopic Surgery Revolution*, or the *Minimally Invasive Surgery Revolution*. Purists will call it the *Minimal Access Surgery Revolution*. Old fashioned surgery required the surgeon to cut open the body of a patient in order to access the internal organs. Surgeons now operate through tiny holes, using a high definition endoscopic camera, and can minimize damage to the external surface of the body; thus, pain is reduced to a minimum.

Surgery for obesity and diabetes is done through tiny holes that cause minimum pain and heal very quickly. One of the holes is always through the umbilicus, and doesn't even cause a scar. The rest are 0.5 cm to 1 cm in diameter, and cause minimal pain. Most patients, nowadays, can immediately get up and walk when they wake up from surgery. The next day, they are usually walking around like normal. I usually require my patients to take a 15-minute walk every 2 hours when they are awake. This helps them to prepare for discharge the following day.

In the bad old days of open surgery, patients generally stayed for 5 to 7 days in hospital. Nowadays, patients stay for 1 to 3 days, with an average of 2 days. They generally sleep a mere 2 nights in hospital.

Pain, nowadays, is measured on a pain analog scale of 1 to 10. Most patients have pain levels of 2 or 3, but some have pain levels of 5 or 6 on the first day. We give analgesics to this group, who may have a lower pain threshold. Generally, they get off injectable analgesics the day after surgery, and only need oral analgesics. The pain gets considerably better the day after surgery, and is usually much better on the second post-operative day.

More than 10 years ago, I had a laparoscopic assisted operation to donate a kidney. The operation was done by keyhole, or minimal access surgery (MAS). However, they needed to make a small incision to remove my kidney. Therefore, I had an opportunity to feel for myself the difference between keyhole surgery and open. When I woke up from the surgery, I felt some pain, but I was happy about that because it meant that I was alive and had survived the operation.

The pain score was about 3 out of 10 at most, and there was no pain unless I moved around. There was no pain when I lay still. The next day, I already forced myself to get up. There was considerable pain in the lower abdominal incision where the kidney was removed, but I hardly even noticed the pain from the keyhole incision they had made to do the surgery. The pain, however, was not severe enough for me to need injectable analgesics, though I was fitted with a pump that allowed me to dose myself if necessary. I never used it. The pain from the incision was bearable—about 5 out of 10. The pain from the small holes was hardly noticeable. The maximum pain came when trying to get out of bed. I soon learnt how to minimize it. First, I would roll to the side, and then I would press a pillow against my abdomen. It hurt much less by getting up in this position, and the pressure from the pillow helped greatly. The following day, I was walking very actively. The next day, I asked to be discharged, and I went out for a good lunch with my ex-wife, so I only spent three days in the hospital after surgery. Within a week, I was back in the OR doing my own operations.

Disability after surgery is now a thing of the past. The downtime, even after relatively major procedures, is now relatively short, especially after MAS. Not making big incisions and cutting open body cavities has made a huge difference to recovery.

In the second half of the 1990s, we took "minimally invasive" one step further, and pioneered mini laparoscopy or needlescopic surgery, together with Michel Gagner and others. It became possible to use even smaller, needle-sized holes to do surgery. Instruments shrank to 2mm or 3mm in diameter, producing hardly any pain and practically no scar. I brought this technology to Brazil, and it was embraced enthusiastically by Gustavo Carvalho, a handsome, young Brazilian surgeon who is now the champion of this technique worldwide.

The next, and probably the biggest fear of going for surgery, is complications of surgery. This is certainly a big psychological obstacle, and will keep many diabetics popping pills and sticking themselves with needles rather than seeking a once and for all reversal or cure of the disease. The fear is primeval and deep seated.

Admittedly, there is a mortality rate and a complication rate from surgery. Both have been dropping drastically over the years, as the technology and the technique of metabolic surgery has improved steadily. Let's take the example of air travel. Airplanes were experimental and highly dangerous at the turn of the 20th century. Some brave souls braved the terrible risk, and this has led to a transport system so safe that few think twice before getting onto a plane and travelling halfway around the world. Yet if one sits down and counts the number of air disasters, one realizes that it is not that uncommon. Recently, one Malaysian Airlines plane disappeared without a trace, and another was shot down by a missile over Ukraine. Malaysian Airlines lost some business, but people continued to fly.

Closer to home, we should consider the operation of coronary artery bypass. This is a truly dangerous operation, where mortality and morbidity is considerable. Nevertheless, patients who have coronary artery disease are quite willing to undergo this rather painful and risky procedure, because they understand the benefits. It would relieve the pain they suffer from, and add years to their life. Eighty percent would get relief from angina pain. Seven percent of patients died at 4 years, compared to 33% in the medically treated group. The operation brought hope of symptom relief and longer life. Patients bought it and were willing to undergo the risky and painful operation to get the benefits. It has been a standard operation for nearly 50 years now.

Metabolic surgery to reverse diabetes, like all surgical procedures, has a mortality and morbidity rate. You know this, and this makes some of you nervous. It is important to remember that almost no activity is risk free. Not doing surgery and reversing your diabetes is also taking a risk! The nonsurgical route exposes you to diabetic complications, which are mostly life threatening or debilitating. It also exposes you to the side effects and dangers of drugs and insulin. On the surface, taking medication may seem simpler and safer than surgery, but over the long term, this becomes untrue; rather, the reverse is true. Over the long term, having surgery to reverse your diabetes actually works out to be less risky. There is about a 1% risk of serious complications when undergoing metabolic surgery. The mortality rate is now down to 0.3%, in data from good centers. In all respects, metabolic surgery is much safer than coronary artery bypass, and the danger is now comparable to laparoscopic gall bladder surgery. The complications are also far less serious, and the pain and hospitalization far less than a CABG.

Despite all the scientific evidence that metabolic surgery is safe, effective, and reproducible, some degree of fear remains in many. In the end, the decision comes down to a cost benefit analysis. You have to weigh the risk with the benefits: what you risk versus what you have to gain.

On the risk side, there is a 0.3% chance of dying, and a 1+% chance of serious complication.

The gain side is enormous:

- If male, 11 years longer life expectancy, and 13 years if female
- 50% reduction in chance of getting cancer
- 50% or more reduction in risk of getting heart disease or stroke
- Reversal of hypertension and high cholesterol in 70% of cases
- Improvement in renal function in those with diabetic nephropathy
- Reversal of fatty liver disease
- More rapid healing of diabetic foot and leg issues
- Improvement in eyesight in those with diabetic retinopathy
- Improved sexual function in both sexes
- Loss of excess weight
- Improvement in overall physical fitness and exercise capacity

If you are a diabetic patient, please add up the sums and see if these benefits are enough to overcome your fear, and put yourself in the hands of your metabolic surgeon to get your problem fixed.

In the field of medicine, fear is a ubiquitous problem. Good medicine requires a change in thinking in the general population, and among doctors as well. Every time something new occurs, like a big scientific breakthrough, it takes time for the new treatment to gain traction. Information has to spread, doctors have to be retrained, and facilities have to be built. Eventually, a successful concept or technology proves itself.

The North America Bariatric Surgery Market has been estimated at USD 589.24 million, in 2016, and is projected to reach USD 1,155 million by 2021, at a CAGR of 11.6% during the forecast period from 2016 to 2021. There are now around 250,000 procedures being done in the USA every year.

Fortunately, the technology for metabolic surgery does not require heavy investment in equipment or resources. However, it does require trained teams, and this does take time to develop.

One other source of fear and weakening of resolve is the misguided advice of the ignorant. There are 3 main sources for such misguided advice. The first of these is the intervention of ignorant friends and relatives. Many of these people would point out the risk of surgery, without balancing this with the wonderful benefits. Many have heard of the anecdotal bad experience or disaster, and emphasize these spectacular events without considering all the smooth, successful cases that had passed unnoticed. The problem is the same as that in the air transport industry. The news plays up the odd crash but does not report the millions of safe and uneventful flights that occur every day. Disaster makes news, and it sticks in the memory much more than the successful and uneventful. Similarly, if a train or a bus gets blown up, it makes headline news and lives in the memory for years or decades, far overshadowing the millions of uneventful bus or train rides that people take every day.

Even more unfortunate is the advice of ignorant or vested members of the medical profession itself. Many doctors still live in the era where it was taught that diabetes is an incurable life-long disease. Many of these doctors do not primarily treat diabetes, but they consider themselves well informed on the subject. They have not kept up with the scientific literature, and are ignorant of the advances that have occurred. In my experience, 90% of my medical colleagues fall into this category. These doctors would blatantly advise the patient that diabetes is incurable and irreversible, and to not waste their time. Sadly, they speak from ignorance.

A second group of doctors are those that know about the amazing efficacy of metabolic surgery, and are afraid and worried about the impact of this development on their own business. When I asked one such doctor why he did not inform his patient that reversal and even cure can be achieved via surgery, he remarked, "We are in the business of selling medication. If we promote the surgical option, how will we make any money?" Another said, "We are not in the business of surgery. We are physicians."

The best people to talk to are those who have undergone the operation, and had their disease reversed and are leading a healthier and better life, free of drugs and injections. Most post-operative patients are very willing to talk about their experience. They are willing to give testimonials on video, social media, or television.

In summary, this is the take-home message if the idea of surgery frightens you:

- Surgery is less painful, more comfortable, and less dangerous than ever before. Downtime is very short.
- Don't listen to anyone who is not an expert on the subject or has vested interest not to cure you. This includes relatives and doctors.
- Do your own research.
- Talk to those who have been reversed or cured.

- Remember that *no surgery* is far more dangerous than surgery.

This is the most important message to keep in mind:

It is more dangerous not to have surgery than to have surgery.

Chapter 11

The Surgery and Aftermath from the Patient's Point of View

Many people view surgery as scary, but in the 21st century, this is much less so. Surgery has never been safer, and the best thing about being in this century is that we have already undergone the minimally invasive revolution.

When I was a young resident, we were encouraged to make big incisions. There used to be a saying: "The bigger the incision, the bigger the surgeon." In the late 1980s, the laparoscopic or Minimally Invasive (MIS) Revolution hit the surgical world. It started with appendectomy and gall bladder resection, but soon spread to the whole gamut of surgical operations. I was fortunate to be one of the pioneers in this revolution, and it swept the whole field of surgery, changing everything.

Patients who used to take many days and even weeks to recover, now go home in one or two days, and are relatively pain free and mobile, even on the first day after the operation. The need for pain killers also dropped substantially.

The experience for a patient undergoing bariatric or metabolic surgery today goes something like this:

There are one or two pre-operative consults, where the patient is assessed for suitability and fitness. This usually takes about 30 minutes, and a battery of blood tests are done. The patient usually has an electrocardiogram, and is scheduled for a gastroscopy, to make sure the stomach holds no surprises like an ulcer or tumor. In 99.9% of cases, the patient would pass these tests. If the ECG shows any abnormality, the patient would require a treadmill ECG and a cardiology consult.

A few days before the surgery, the surgeon would do a pre-operative consult, where he will explain the risks, the post-operative course, the post-operative diet regime, the complications, and the vitamin requirement after the surgery. During this time, a consent would be taken and a patient advisory signed, to make sure the patient understands everything. Questions would be taken.

On the day of the operation, one or two hours before, you would need to check in, and come with an empty stomach, having taken no food after midnight the previous day, and no drink for 6 hours before the surgery. Essential medication would continue to be consumed. If the patient is on aspirin or platelet blockers for his heart problem or stroke, then these must be omitted for at least a week.

The surgeon would usually come before the surgery, to see that the patient is calm and well, and to answer any last questions. Some lighthearted reassurance would be given that everything will be fine. The anesthetist will then brief you. He will take an anesthetic history and run through the small risks of putting you to sleep. He will set an intravenous line and then put you to sleep. When you wake up—which of course feels like a few seconds—everything will be over, and you will be in the recovery room waiting for transport to your own room. In 99% of cases, there is no need for observation in the intensive care unit. This may be necessary if you have a serious pre-existing medical problem (e.g., abnormal heart rhythms).

Immediately after surgery, you may be required to not take anything orally, but if everything went super well, ice chips or sips of water may

The Surgery and Aftermath from the Patient's Point of View

be allowed. You will be on pain killers and anti-nausea medication, but the surgeon would have given you nerve blocks during the operation, so you will not feel much pain from the tiny puncture wounds in the abdomen. You may have an abdominal drain and be on foot or leg pumps to avoid deep vein thrombosis. Hydration will be totally intravenous for the first day, and you will also have 8 hourly blood sugar tests. During the day of surgery, and the first night, the blood sugar tends to be high because of the sugar in the intravenous fluids. You will be encouraged to walk to the toilet, should you need to go. There may be some nausea, abdominal cramps, and reflux the first night, which will be controlled by medication. The first night is usually a little uncomfortable. I usually sedate the patients well, so that the night will pass quickly.

You will see a dramatic improvement in all aspects the next day. Pain, colic, nausea, and reflux would all suddenly improve dramatically. Most patients feel completely well. The blood sugar and blood pressure would also show dramatic improvement. You will be taken off all fluids containing sugar, and your intravenous drip would be switched to normal saline. You may come off insulin and still maintain normal blood sugars, or require very small doses. Patients previously on regular insulin might see a dramatic drop in their insulin requirement, or even get off it. It is not uncommon to see some patients get off all drugs and insulin on the very next day after the surgery. You will be encouraged to take 15-minute walks every 2 hours, and to take 30 to 50cc of clear fluids, like water or plain tea, every hour. The amount of oral fluids will be increased gradually. Usually, patients will be surprised at their level of comfort and mobility. Most patients can even walk up a flight of stairs, and walk round the block outside if the weather permits.

The morning after the surgery, the doctor will start you on oral fluids. If you are diabetic, it is best to start with water or plain tea. You will be taught to sip your drink a small mouthful at a time, let it go down, and see if there is any hold up or pain. If fluids go down easily, and there is no pain or vomiting, the recovery will usually progress smoothly. Fluids are slowly increased over the next days. If the operation is for obesity or hypertension, then the choice of fluids is more varied. Gassy drinks are best avoided during this period, as gas retention can be quite annoying.

The three most common early post-operative complications are anastomotic leak, bleeding, or deep vein thrombosis. All three are very uncommon. Leak is the most feared, and this is usually heralded by severe abdominal pain. In my practice, I always leave an abdominal drain so that leak can be detected and more easily managed. In modern practice, leaks are often managed conservatively by drainage, and either stenting or inserting a feeding tube, distal to the site of the leak. This seems to give the better outcome than repeat surgery, either laparoscopic or open. Leaks from sleeve resections are, on the whole, best treated this way. Leaks would of course prolong your hospital stay.

Bleeding is even less common. This can be bleeding into the abdominal cavity or bleeding into the bowel, which then presents with black stools or vomiting of fresh or digested blood. Most times, the bleeding is very minor and stops on its own without surgical or endoscopic intervention. Bleeding is best avoided, rather than treated, by meticulous attention during the surgery to check for bleeding, and stop even the smallest amount of bleeding.

Deep vein thrombosis happens because patients are obese. It is also more likely to happen to Caucasians rather than Asians. As usual, it is best avoided rather than treated. Prophylaxis include calf and foot pumps, compression stockings, and light anticoagulation with low molecular weight heparin. Anticoagulation is a two- edged sword, as too much can cause bleeding. Asians generally don't need it unless super obese. If it happens, despite all preventative measures, anticoagulation will usually resolve the problem.

The Surgery and Aftermath from the Patient's Point of View

On the second day, the patient will increase the amount of fluids taken orally each time, and will be totally off intravenous fluids. The drain will be removed. More walking is encouraged, and the patient gets a shower, a dressing change, and dresses for home. Most often, the blood pressure and blood sugar will already be normal, without medication. This occurs even with insulin-dependent, type 2 diabetics. The time to go back to work depends more on the patient's occupation rather than on the restriction imposed by the surgery itself. The Russian Minister of Finance flew back to Moscow, from Nizhny Novgorod, and went back to work on the third day after the surgery. Russians are, on the whole, somewhat robust. One employee of the National University of Singapore's engineering department took the opportunity to take 2 months of hospitalization leave! In general, most patients can go back to work within 5 days to a week.

You can also return to physical activity relatively quickly. All my patients can walk around on the first day, and can climb stairs. One governor from Russia swam in the famous sky pool, at Marina Bay Sands in Singapore, 3 days after laparoscopic gastric sleeve resection. An Indonesian multi-millionaire was back on the golf course, on the 10th day after surgery.

On the whole, patients who undergo metabolic surgery can expect their physical exercise tolerance to improve markedly. After having the surgery, one Indian hotelier who, before surgery, could not even walk for 7 minutes, lost 80kg and could run for 45 minutes. After a 15-minute rest, he could run for another 45 minutes. An English school teacher could not even swim one lap of a swimming pool before surgery, but could do 30 laps, 2 months after surgery. Improvement in neuropathy and diabetic foot infections also means that patients are much more mobile after the diabetes is reversed. A minimum of 150 minutes of exercise a week is encouraged.

In terms of diet, the patient has to accept a one-month transition from fluids to semi-solids, to full diet. During the first week, we usually recommend strictly fluids and clear soups of broth. The fluids should not contain any sugar. In the second week, the patients may transition to yogurt and very runny, soft-boiled eggs. After two weeks, the patient may have a soft diet consisting of purees and thin soups. Steamed fish may be allowed, as is minced meat or chicken. Vegetables should be pureed. This will continue for another 2 weeks. After that, normal diet is allowed, but the patient is encouraged to eat slowly and chew well. The best diet for the diabetic post-surgery would be low in carbohydrates and sugar. The modern trend toward a ketogenic diet is ideal.

A frequent question from patients is whether they can eat like a normal person. This is a loaded question, because their previous diet was usually unhealthy, and it could not be considered a normal, healthy diet. I think the answer is that they can go back to a normal, healthy diet. The emphasis is on the word, *healthy*.

Going back on a high carbohydrate, high sugar diet, which caused their diabetes in the first place, is one of the ways to get a recurrence of the disease. What surgery does is reset you back to before you had the diabetes, and now you have a responsibility to try a different lifestyle so that you can avoid getting the disease again. Most patients can make a permanent recovery from the disease.

This is not the same as trying to reverse your diabetes by diet and exercise alone, without surgery. Doing that is really difficult and is rarely sustainable. The regime is far less strict once surgery has been done.

Finally, we need to discuss the issue of vitamins. Metabolic surgery does have one small downside: Vitamin absorption is generally decreased, and vitamin supplements are required. The normal regime is multivitamins, B complex, B12, iron, and calcium. Once a year, patients should check their vitamin levels for deficiency. The commonest deficiency is Vitamin B12, which leads to fatigue and tiredness; and calcium and Vitamin D deficiency, which can lead to decreased bone density.

In summary, the surgical and post-surgical experiences are remarkable for comfort, safety, and speedy recovery. Most patients expect a painful, medieval experience but are pleasantly surprised that it's more like something out of *Star Trek*. Technology has really come a long way since Theodor Billroth first performed stomach surgery in the 1880s, at the Allgemeine Krankenhaus in Vienna.

Even more astounding is the quick reversal of objective parameters. Blood sugar drops promptly to normal levels within days, and blood pressure as well. Most times, patients come off medication within days after the surgery. The most spectacular recovery I have seen was with the wife of a 3-star general from Indonesia. The husband was the chief of the Indonesian equivalent of the American CIA. Her blood sugar dropped to normal, one day after surgery, without medication or insulin, and she became one of the most active advocates of metabolic surgery in Jakarta.

How do patients do long term?

This was the subject of an 18-year Swedish study on what happens to patients who had undergone bariatric surgery. They found a 50% reduction in cardiovascular risk, which means that they reduced their risk of heart attack and stroke by 50%. There was also improvement in the risk for peripheral artery disease. The cancer incidence in this group was also reduced by 50%, to a level that approached the normal population.

Long-term follow-up of the diabetes showed that in 5 years, 65% of patients remained non-diabetic, and 35% recurred. The same Swedish study, however, showed that even in those that recurred, the reduction in cardiovascular risk and cancer risk was sustained. This is truly remarkable!

Chapter 12

Prediabetes – Don't Ignore It

Most diabetics pass through a stage of prediabetes and may not even know it. Prediabetes is defined the same mathematically as diabetes. If you have a HbA1C of 5.7% to 6.4%, you are pre-diabetic. The minute you reach 6.5%, you have diabetes. In terms of fasting sugar levels, it is 100mg/dl to 125 mg/dl. If you are thinking metric, it is 5.5mmole/l to 6.7mmole/l. Another index is a 2-hour, oral glucose tolerance test result of 7.7mmole/l.

There are probably as many pre-diabetics as there are diabetics. No one knows for sure, because 80% to 90% are undiagnosed. An estimated 33.9% of US adults, aged 18 or older (84.1 million), had prediabetes in 2015. Nearly half of those over 65 have it.

Only 11.6% know that they have it. It is generally a silent disease. Most are totally asymptomatic, but some have early symptoms of diabetes, like thirst, frequent urination, blurring of vision, and feeling tired. If you are always feeling tired, you should have your blood sugar checked.

Predisposing factors are:

- Gestational diabetes: 50% eventually become diabetic.
- Polycystic ovarian disease.
- Race: American Indians and Pacific Islanders have the highest incidence. In Asia, it is the Indians and the Malaysians.

- Obesity: definite co-relation.
- Hyperlipidemia: raised LDL, total cholesterol, and triglycerides, and low HDL.
- Lack of exercise and sedentary lifestyle.
- Over 45 years of age.
- Having a waist size of more than 40 inches (100 cm) in males, and 35 inches (89cm) in women.
- A previous raised blood sugar level.
- Heart disease.
- Raised insulin levels.

If you have prediabetes, you have a 25% to 30% chance of becoming diabetic in 3 to 5 years, and more than a 40% lifetime chance of becoming a diabetic.

This is a condition you cannot ignore, and you must do everything to reverse it.

How best to reverse the condition, however, requires making some decisions.

The Conventional Way

Most professionals, myself included, believe that some lifestyle changes should be the starting point. So, the following measures should be immediately started:

- Lose weight; even 5 or 10 kg would make a difference.
- Exercise for at least 30 minutes, 3 times a week, but preferably 5 times.
- Stop smoking.
- Treat the hypertension.
- Eat more healthily.

The diet should consist of:

- Whole grains
- No sweet drinks, and no sugar in tea or coffee
- Good fats such as olive oil and vegetable oil, and less saturated fats and fried foods
- Nuts and seeds
- Protein, especially poultry and fish, and less red meat.

There is now a school that believes that early introduction of hypoglycemic drugs may be the way to go, but this is controversial and not universally accepted. Drugs are expensive and have side effects, and the pros and cons must be carefully weighed. Going on drugs would immediately tie you to medical supervision and attending regular follow-ups at clinics. Pharmaceutical companies would of course be delighted. The question is whether insurance would pay for it.

Metformin, at the moment, is the only drug approved for treatment of prediabetes. As it is relatively cheap and safe, there is probably no harm in taking metformin; but the question is, is it necessary?

There is, however, a big need to reverse this condition; otherwise, diabetes is inevitable.

What about surgery for the pre-diabetic?

Almost all morbidly obese people are pre-diabetic. Obese people are 80 times more likely to develop diabetes than those with a BMI of 22 or less. Women with a BMI of 30, have 28 times greater risk of developing diabetes. For those with a BMI of 35 and above, it is 93 times. Obesity itself is a pre-diabetic condition. Surgery would therefore, in this group, be directed at the obesity rather than at the diabetes.

If a pre-diabetic is morbidly obese, bariatric surgery would reverse the prediabetes easily. The best time to reverse diabetes is always early rather than late.

What should an obese pre-diabetic do?

First of all, try every means you know of to lose weight. Go on a healthy diet of vegetables, nuts, seeds, beans, and fresh fruit. Reduce refined carbohydrates. Exercise vigorously. If you fail to lose weight despite these measures, then seriously consider a gastric sleeve resection. A one-hour procedure could solve all your problems, bringing your weight down rapidly, reversing your pre-diabetic condition, and getting your HbA1c below 5.7%.

What about the non-obese pre-diabetic?

I would eat healthily and exercise like the above. Even a small weight loss might make a difference. If this doesn't work, and you become diabetic, with a HbA1C of 6.5% or higher, then your choices are medication or surgery. If you want to reverse your diabetes long term, surgery should be done sooner rather than later, as the results are far better when the surgery is done earlier.

I would not be too concerned about weight criteria for surgery, unless you are very thin, as the criteria keep changing over time anyway. Normal weight diabetics do not become very thin after metabolic surgery. They lose a few kilograms but generally don't get into an overly underweight situation. The reversal chances are 77% to 80%. There are more and more publications on low BMI metabolic surgery, which all show reasonable results.

In summary, if you are pre-diabetic, the first thing to do is to change your diet to a low carbohydrate, low sugar diet, and try your best to lose weight. If you are already obese, then surgery becomes a good option, as you will solve both the weight and the pre-diabetes problem simultaneously. Otherwise, the other option is lifelong medication, with all the attendant downsides. If your HbA1C remains at 6.4% or below, it is probably not necessary to go on long-term medication.

Weight loss options are many, and there are non-surgical expedients, such as the gastric balloon, which are effective at least in the short term.

Chapter 13

Why Obesity Must Be Reversed

If you are overweight or obese, it is imperative that you try to get back to normal weight. Any excuse you give not to do so is hazardous to your life and health, and is sheer denial.

- Your life will be shortened by 11 years for men, and 13 years for women. Bariatric surgery has been statistically shown to extend your life by these amounts.
- You will have double the risk of heart disease and stroke.
- You will double your risk of getting cancer.
- Your excess weight will put extra stress on your spine and joints, leading to backache and arthritis.
- You get sleep apnoea, which can lead to dying in your sleep.
- You get reflux, which can cause cancer of the lower oesophagus.
- You will have a higher chance of getting gallstones.
- Obesity increases the risk of diabetes hypertension and high cholesterol.
- Obesity leads to fatty liver, which can lead to liver failure.
- Obese people are two times more likely to have a stroke.
- Obesity increases the risk of asthma.
- There is reduced sperm count in men, and infertility in women.

The exponential increase in obesity in recent decades parallels the steep rise in the incidence of diabetes. In the USA, 85% of diabetics are overweight or obese, and the two conditions are increasing in tandem. For every 20% of body weight over the ideal, the chances of diabetes doubles.

In Asia, people have more body fat in relation to their BMI, so diabetes occurs at a much lower BMI. A study in China showed that men with a BMI of 23.7 had 25% body fat, and females with a BMI of only 21.2, already had 32% body fat.

Body fat is therefore a stronger correlation with diabetic risk than with BMI. Nevertheless, there is no controversy that the higher your BMI, the greater your risk for diabetes.

It is therefore imperative for obese people to lose weight however they can, if they want to avoid diabetes; and for diabetics, who are already overweight or obese, to do the same if they want to get a better control over their blood sugar.

Chapter 14

Politics and Economics in the Diabetes World

The Interest of the Doctors

Why don't doctors tell diabetic patients about metabolic surgery, which can reverse their disease? This is a question I get from almost every patient I speak to about reversing or curing their disease. After some research of the problem, I came up with this long list of reasons: Very many doctors still have not heard about it. Many doctors only follow updates in their own specialty. General practitioners have too many talks to choose from, and may not have gone to talks on this subject. I would estimate that 70% to 80% of GPs haven't heard about it.

Endocrinologists and diabetologists know about this option but generally would definitely not tell their patients about it. They see it as a threat to their practice.

- They don't benefit from promoting reversal or cure.
- They can't do it themselves and can never learn it.
- They lose the patient once he/she is reversed or cured.
- They suffer financial loss.

Many doctors make money from not reversing or curing the disease. Money comes from drugs, blood tests, consultations, and the treatment of complications from the disease.

- Kidney specialists make money from treating diabetic kidney disease. Think of how much money is made doing dialysis.
- Heart specialists make money from heart disease, which is secondary to diabetes.
- Neurologists make money from stroke and nerve problems.
- Skin specialists make money from skin problems secondary to diabetes.
- Eye doctors make money from treating diabetic retinopathy.

In summary, every doctor is making money from not curing diabetes. Drug companies have no interest in curing diabetes.

The government does not want to pay for the operations, so they don't promote it.

The only person who benefits from reversing or curing diabetes is the diabetic. He benefits hugely. Just ask anyone who has been cured.

Many patients also ask about the Hippocratic Oath. Shouldn't doctors put the patient's interest above their own? Generally, doctors do put the patient's interest first, if it is possible, but you must understand the harsh environment of medical practice in today's world.

In many countries, the income from the sale of drugs constitutes a large source of revenue for the general practitioners and the endocrinologists. Curing the disease would result in a severe loss of income. It is far easier for them to ignore any new developments, than to jeopardize their secure, ongoing income. They practice in a high cost, high risk environment, and life is not easy for them either. Unfortunately, this is a technology they can't benefit from. Both GPs and endocrinologists cannot easily convert to bariatric surgeons. They can't benefit from curing you.

Well, this is not entirely true. A very smart GP or diabetic specialist would partner with a bariatric surgeon, and form diabetic centers offering all options. This is the best way to move with the times and not suffer financial loss.

What about the interest of other specialists downstream? Many doctors in other specialties make a lot of money dealing with the complications of chronic diseases, and they would also suffer if the problem got solved at the root. Patients would then not need their services, and the impact on them would be great.

Cardiologists, for instance, would have much less coronary artery disease to treat. There would be far fewer stenting procedures. Heart surgeons would have less coronary artery bypass grafts to do.

There would be much fewer kidney failures. Kidney specialists would have fewer patients. Dialysis centers would suffer. Kidney transplant surgeons would see fewer transplant patients.

Orthopedic surgeons would see less diabetic foot problems, and do less amputations. Vascular surgeons would see less peripheral arterial disease, and do fewer procedures.

Eye specialists would have fewer diabetic retinopathies to treat, and fewer operations to do. Skin specialists would see less diabetic-related skin problems. Neurologists would have less diabetic neuropathy to treat, and fewer stroke patients to manage.

Nutritionists and dieticians would have less work. The millions of people claiming to be able to reverse diabetes by special diets and supplements, would suffer as well.

You can see why metabolic surgery is so unpopular in the medical community. Everyone is making a living out of not curing disease. A one-off solution is thus everyone's nightmare.

That is, except for one person—the diabetic patient.

The bar to becoming a metabolic and bariatric surgeon is very high, and is insurmountable to most doctors. The doctor would first have to qualify as a surgeon, then an upper gastrointestinal surgeon, and then a bariatric and metabolic surgeon. For a non-surgeon, this would take a minimum of eight years. Hardly anyone, not already a surgeon, can spare the time. So, unfortunately, for most doctors dealing with diabetes, they can't convert easily to exploit this development.

Doctors who treat diabetes are used to being in control, and are used to selling drugs and insulin. They are not at all keen to pass control on to anyone else. Traditionally, diabetes is a medical problem. It has been so since 1922. Now the surgeons have an overwhelmingly superior technology, and doctors are not sure how to react to this.

The Drug Companies

It is a formidable task to get a drug FDA approved. First, millions have to be spent in research. After that, the approval process requires several phases of animal and then human trials. The whole process will cost many millions of USD, and sometimes billions.

Drug companies thus need to make the money back somehow, and also show a profit for their shareholders. The best cash cows are drugs that control chronic diseases but do not cure.

There are 450 to 500 million diabetics in the world, and drugs alone are a trillion dollar business. Pharmaceutical companies are very, very rich, and their strategy is to keep you dependent on their products for life. That is their business model. Curing chronic diseases is totally not on their agenda.

Let's look at some of the figures. In the USA, the average cost of medical expenses per year, for a diabetic, is $13,700. On the diabetes itself, $7,900 is spent. People who have diabetes spend 2.3 times more than the average person.

Spending on diabetes in the USA alone, per year, is $245 billion USD. If you are on insulin, in the USA, you will spend $450 per month on the average.

The economic cost of diabetes has increased 26% in the last 5 years. The lifetime cost of treating type 2 diabetes, broken down by age group, would be:

25 to 44 years – $ 124,700
45 to 54 years – $ 106,200
55 to 64 years – $ 84,000
>65 years   – $ 54,700

Contrast this to the average cost of surgery in the USA, of $20,000 to $30,000. After that, you save not only on diabetes medication but also on medicine for hypertension and high cholesterol.

It is no surprise that the pharmaceutical industry is less that enamored by the introduction of bariatric and metabolic surgery.

You will notice that even though all the drug companies advertise heavily in the USA, which is one of the only countries in the world that can do this, they are strangely silent about all curative options.

In conclusion, the pharmaceutical industry cannot benefit from curing your problem; thus, they have no interest in curing you whatsoever. This seems cynical, but they are not in business to cure people but to make money. They have shareholders to answer to.

Medical Tech Companies

Then there are the many medical tech companies that make devices like glucometers, insulin pumps, monitors, etc. These companies also stand to lose if you get cured. There would be no more need for glucose measuring machines, test strips, swabs, monitoring devices, insulin pumps, etc. Of course, there would still be the type 1 diabetes market, which isn't going anywhere soon.

The other group of companies make equipment for laparoscopic gastric surgery. These make energy devices for surgery, like the harmonic shears or ultracision, and laparoscopic staplers and trocars. These companies stand to benefit from more surgery, and are the commercial entities that are willing to promote bariatric and metabolic surgery. Many large medical giants make both types of equipment, and they are in a dilemma as to which one to promote more. They either shoot themselves in one foot or the other.

Governments and Health Authorities

Surprisingly, governments and health authorities stand to gain in the long term. An aging population and an exponential increase in chronic diseases, in most developed countries, is threatening to overwhelm health budgets everywhere. Infrastructure expansion cannot keep pace, and the budget will never be enough. Increasing taxes is unpopular and may lead to election losses.

If the prevalence of diabetes doubles, the number of complications from diabetes will double. The numbers will increase. This will double the cost of health care. Governments cannot afford to let this happen. To reduce this, they need to spend money now; but they are reluctant to do this, because this needs diversion of funds from other areas such as, perhaps, defense. Our government has decided to try and do this the cheap way, which of course doesn't work.

Their approach is to push back the responsibility to the citizen, and declare war on diabetes, and get everyone to eat more healthily and exercise. Of course, this is just window dressing and won't even dent the problem. When has just telling people to live a healthier life ever got anyone to comply? Historically, that is just not going to happen.

People live unhealthy lives because society is structured in such a way that people work all the time and have no time for exercise, and unhealthy food is far cheaper than healthy food. Besides, it often tastes better and is more convenient and accessible.

Curing diabetes would save billions, but you may have to spend billions in the short term to save trillions in the long term. Governments, looking only to the next year's budget, would probably not commit to funding metabolic surgery. They will regret this in the long term when they have to pay for coronary stenting, cancer surgery, chemotherapy, kidney disease, management of stroke, diabetic foot treatment, amputations, laser treatment for diabetic retinopathy, and many more.

The correct policy for governments would be to send as many diabetics as will go for metabolic surgery. It's both curative and preventive. Under most systems, this would save billions and even trillions of dollars in the long run, save many lives, and stave off a huge amount of disease load in the future. This requires a brave and far-sighted health minister and government.

A smart government would be in favor of a cure.

Unfortunately, this is not the reality. Most health authorities are offering metabolic surgery but are making it super hard for patients to access it. They introduce many barriers, and they make the patient pass many gateways. For example, there must be a compulsory period of diet and exercise. There are inflexible BMI criteria. There are many levels of doctors to see, even before they reach a bariatric surgeon, and most of these levels are trying their best to discourage the patient. Insurance companies also put up their own barriers, which are designed to delay or reject.

This forces many into the private sector to get their diabetes fixed.

There are several other options that governments can consider, which may have some effect. The tax on sugar, by the UK, is one good example. The people who insist on increasing their risk of getting diabetes, by taking large amounts of sugar and sweet drinks, should help to pay for the health expenditure that their behavior will undoubtedly cause.

Another idea I like is to use tax incentives to encourage weight control. Individuals with BMIs in the obese range should have a slightly higher income tax penalty, and those that maintain their BMI in the normal range should be rewarded with a tax cut by an equal amount. In a socialist system, I think this is fair, as the obese would presumably be prone to diabetes and hypertension, and therefore use more resources. They should thus pay more taxes. This would be an added incentive to keep slim. It would also be further incentive to have bariatric surgery, if one cannot achieve the correct BMI by lifestyle change. We need brave governments to enact these measures.

Insurance Companies

The predicament of insurance companies is similar to that of governments: Spend now or spend much more later. To their credit, insurance companies are beginning to see this slowly, and are more and more willing to pay for the procedures to reverse or cure diabetes. Insurance companies are not all the same, though. Some are more advanced in their thinking, and some are less so. Insurance executives, like politicians, are often prone to short-term rather than long-term thinking. Thinking long term, the decision to cure is a no-brainer. The savings, long term, are tremendous.

Insurance companies do have one extra line of defense. Unlike governments who are responsible for the health of the whole population, insurance companies are only responsible to look after their customers, and they have the power to choose their customers. They simply refuse to insure all those with pre-existing disease, like diabetes and hypertension. That way, they lower their risk and ensure that most of their customers would remain relatively well, and not develop medical problems that would be expensive for them. It's a smart policy on their part but leaves lots of people uninsurable. This was the problem that President Barack Obama was trying to address when he introduced Obamacare. Unfortunately, his term ended before he could really make it work. In the USA, no one has worked out how to solve this problem yet. The idea of universal health care, mooted by some Democratic presidential candidates for the coming 2020 elections, would cost an immense amount of money, and it is uncertain where that money would come from. The problem of diabetes is going to overwhelm the health budgets of most countries. There is one small light at the end of the tunnel. Metabolic surgery is now recognized to reverse or cure diabetes in many cases. After 3 to 5 years, a former diabetic would have normal blood sugars and HbA1c results, without insulin or medication. This means that he or she could successfully get health insurance. We have already seen this happen. Some insurance companies are already putting this into practice, and some of my long-term patients have got insured.

Another healthy development in this field is that some patients, who had insurance before they developed the disease and had the surgery, were able to upgrade their insurance policy for more coverage, without any penalties attributable to their previous diabetic state.
In the pipeline now are some insurance companies willing to insure diabetics on the condition they had metabolic surgery, and on the proviso that they continue to maintain their policy post-surgery, for a fixed number of years. These policies would presumably be more expensive than those targeted at the population with no pre-existing disease. Insurance programs that don't make money cannot survive.

Perspective of the Diabetic Patient

For the patient, the decision is a no-brainer. If you have not yet come to the correct conclusion by now, of what is the best course of action, then you probably are resigned to have an incurable disease, with all its attendant complications. Many patients are like ostriches with their heads buried in the sand. They don't have a problem yet, so they think things will always be the same. The statistics clearly show this to be false.

Once you have a stroke or a heart attack, or you get cancer, or you end up on dialysis, then you would really wish that you had paid more attention to the science.

In short, most diabetics, unless they are very mild, will be better off seeking remission or cure. The main problem will be how to pay for it.

If you have adequate insurance coverage, there is no problem. You can get the cost of surgery totally covered. If you have spare cash around, you would be wise to use it to get yourself cured.

I once spent a long time talking to a rich man from Bangladesh. He was obese, with both hypertension and type 2 diabetes, and was eminently curable. A gastric sleeve resection would have entirely solved his problem. He balked at the price. It would cost about 32,000 (23,500 USD) Singapore dollars to totally fix his health issues. He would be back to normal weight, and his diabetes and hypertension would be gone. He never came back to me. I heard from his friend that two days later, he bought a $35,000 Rolex watch, and then flew back to his country. One day, he will be watching his remaining life tick away on his luxurious watch, while lying in a hospital bed dying from cancer, heart disease, or kidney failure, half paralyzed from a stroke. Don't you think he would have been wiser to fix his health rather than spend money on an expensive watch that he won't even be able to take to the next life?

For those who are not so wealthy, and with no insurance, there are still options. One can get a loan, charge part of the amount to your credit card, borrow from family, relatives, or good friends, or raise money on the internet. One of my prospective patients, from the USA, actually did the last one on the list.

Finally, there is the option of medical tourism. There are many countries where the operation can be done much more cheaply than the USA and Singapore, which are really the two most expensive places to get it done. In Qatar, the operation is done free of charge, but you must be a Qatari citizen. Many people, from the USA, get it done in Mexico.

I have spent the last 5 years creating medical tourism opportunities in cheaper centers around the world. In my company's international network, we can do it for 15,000 USD, in Shanghai, China; and 12,000 USD, in Yekaterinburg, Russia. In both places, we have state-of-the-art facilities and top-class teams.

Unfortunately, even this amount is unaffordable for many people in the world. I do think that those who can afford it should get it done, so that scarce state resources can go to the lower income citizens.

In this section, I have endeavored to show how complicated the political and economic dynamics of the diabetes problem has become in the world. One thing remains clear: If you are suffering from diabetes, your best course of action is to get it attended to as soon as possible. Just like cancer, the longer you wait, the harder it will be to cure your disease. Reverse your diabetes as soon as possible. There are many options to help you overcome the problem of financing your surgery.

Chapter 15

The Road to Reversing Diabetes
– My Personal Journey

I became a doctor because I really wanted to make a difference to the science of medicine, and make a breakthrough that would benefit a large number of people. I wanted to make an impact at the macro level, though I soon learnt that in order to do that, you had to learn to cure the individual patient, and produce good outcomes for each and every patient.

As a child, my passion was classical music and the piano. I could afford to spend a lot of time on this because I was good at studying and taking exams, and that left me a lot of time to concentrate on music. At one point, early in high school, I was a member of 4 different orchestras, in addition to taking piano and oboe lessons, and playing in a bagpipe band. I gave my first piano concert at the age of 9, and also went on television to play the piano. One thing music taught me was to be meticulous and to be error free. This was also important in surgery, where the consequences of mistakes are grave. In both fields, one strives for zero error; but in both fields, this was not an easy goal. At 16, I entered a nationwide, interschool television science quiz. The teams were the best science students in every top Singapore school. My team, from Anglo Chinese School, which was the premier school at that time in 1972, won the first prize, and I answered the last winning question in the finals when we were tied neck and neck with our rival finalist. I still remember the final question: "How many spark plugs are there in a 6-cylinder diesel engine?" Do you know the correct answer? It's a trick question. The answer is *none*. There are no spark plugs in a diesel engine. We won by one question, and I became a child celebrity. That year, I finished the GCE O levels among 7 individuals with the top score in the whole country. I tied for top place in my school.

The choice to continue was obvious. I wanted to do science, and pre-medical was the obvious choice, as it was between that and pre-engineering. I never regretted that decision, which was heavily influenced by my father. He always wanted to become a doctor but could never afford it, and the closest he got was as a medical orderly in the British Army, in the Second World War, fighting the Japanese in the Battle of Singapore. After the fall of Singapore, he was nearly caught and executed, but he survived by hiding among criminals in Outram Road Prison. Thirty-five thousand young male citizens were brought to the beach at Changi and machine gunned. A few escaped to tell the tale, and there were war crime tribunals in retribution after the war.

However, I digress. The last two years of high school in our country are called pre-university. I pursued the pre-medical curriculum, comprising of biology, chemistry, physics, mathematics, and of course, English. During the two years, my school won almost all the music competitions nationally, and also all the science competitions. I participated in all these events, most significantly the national chemistry competition and the science fair, where I led our chemistry project to victory and the top prize.

At the end of the two years, I received the President's Scholarship. It was awarded at the presidential palace—the Istana—by Dr. Benjamin Sheares, our second president, who before politics was a gynecologist. He was a most interesting gentleman, who had delivered the children of every important family in our country.

The scholarship led to medical school, which I chose to do in Singapore; and the Singapore government was kind enough to pay all my tuition and room and board, plus a small allowance for books. It was generous. Singapore University had a very good faculty at that time, which was probably one of the best in Asia but certainly not yet world class. It was a respectable medical school with fine traditions and a very rigorous work ethic. It was certainly not a party school. It was serious. Its successor, the National University of Singapore, is now ranked 26th worldwide, and first in Asia.

Nevertheless, I took two years to find my feet, as I was madly in love for the first two years, with one of my brilliant and attractive classmates. My academic career got back on track the third year after a traumatic break-up. I topped the last two years, and graduated at the top of my class with a clutch of medals and prizes. This, of course, put me into the best possible position of choosing where to do my postgraduate training. I was first priority on everyone's list, so I could choose wherever I wanted to go for my internship. With an academic career in mind, I stuck to the university, of course, and chose to do my rotations in general surgery, medicine, and pediatrics.

I loved surgery right from the start. It was love at first sight. The glamour for me, in a doctor's life, was all about the operating room. That's where you actually got to take a personal hand in fixing the patient's problem. It was up close and personal. It was romantic, technical, artistic, and scientific. It was everything that gave meaning to life and to work.

After internship, came a stint in the army, as a captain and a medical officer. The life of an "officer and a gentleman" suited me, and I always had fantasies about the military, which would play out gradually over the years. It included a stint in Taiwan, with the officer cadets and some exciting war games. After the military, came residency, so it was back to general surgery, then orthopedics and cardiac surgery. They were all really kick-ass assignments. In orthopedics, I was attached to

Prof. Robert Pho, who was a world famous microsurgeon who could reattach fingers and limbs. Working under him, I had the chance to learn some microsurgery, and operate with a microscope. There was one memorable night when a small child came with an almost amputated large toe, and I managed to reattach it, and it survived. Here was also my first introduction to the horrors and ravages of diabetes, as I had to do every type of amputation of gangrenous toes, feet, and legs. This was one of the commonest procedures we had to do in an orthopedic unit, and also the most unpleasant. The results were sad cripples who seldom lived long subsequently.

My cardiac surgery posting was a real thrill. To me, this type of surgery was like going to space. You could stop a heart, fix it, and then restart it while the patient was living off a machine. At that time, it felt like science fiction. Literally, it was like the *Star Trek* mission, "to boldly go where no man has gone before." My flirtation with heart surgery started when I was a third-year student, when I had the opportunity to be assigned to a heart surgeon as my personal tutor. He was flamboyant, wore his hair long, drove a sports car, and sported a sexy mistress and a bevy of beautiful Persian cats. His first task was to educate his students on the joys of cheese and wine. What really impressed me was that he took me—a third-year medical student—to the OR, sliced open the patient's chest, put them on bypass, opened the heart, and invited me to put my fingers into a living heart to feel the mitral valve! Of course, I was impressed into the next galaxy. There was little chance that I would be anything else other than a surgeon after that.

My boss in the cardiac surgery unit was the opposite. He was soft spoken, extremely conservative, and the opposite of flamboyant. He ran a tight ship and kept his residents and fellows on a tight leash. He was super careful. No doubt, he was also an excellent surgeon, but glamour was never his forte. I was grateful, though, to the young fellows in the department, who taught me a great deal. I learnt to open the chest, prepare peripheral veins for coronary artery bypass grafts (CABG), and put a patient on heart-lung bypass—basically to hook them up to a life support machine. Those were useful skills, which proved applicable even though I migrated back to general surgery.

Here, too, I perceived once again the root of all evil, which was, and still is, diabetes. About 40% of patients with ischemic heart disease were diabetic. It was not difficult to postulate that the metabolic problem of blood sugar control had some causal effect in narrowing blood vessels and interfering with the blood supply to the heart.

I found heart surgery to be an amazing field, except for one thing. The politics were frightful. The cardiac surgeon had no direct access to patients, and his success failure and popularity depended totally on the relationship with the cardiologist, who called all the shots. The cardiologists are the ones to decide who should go for surgery and which surgeon gets to do the case. The surgeon was, therefore, just like a technician, with no management function other than a pair of hands to do a job. I felt sorry for the cardiac surgeon, who has trained for so many years and has acquired so much expertise, to be put into such a position.

There will always be a rivalry between the surgeon and the physician. Historically, the physician is the scholar and the scientist, and the surgeon a mere workman. The physician is the thinker, and the surgeon a mere pair of hands, no more important than a barber or a carpenter. Today, the situation has changed. The surgeon knows just as much as the physician, and can do everything the physician can do. If he wants to, he can master all the drugs at the physician's disposal. On the other hand, the physician can never go to the operating room and personally intervene and fix the patient like the surgeon can. Yet in certain fields, the physician, using the politics of control, maintains his dominance. I find this situation totally unacceptable. Thus, I wanted to go into a field where I alone could control patient flow. I needed a specialty where the patient would seek me out directly, bypassing the physician middleman. I didn't want to be a mere pilot. I wanted to be captain of the ship. I wanted to be mission control as well. That's when I decided to go back to general surgery.

The ritual for becoming a surgeon in those days required a trip to the mother country, England, or more correctly, the United Kingdom, to be blessed by the Royal Colleges, and conferred the exalted title of Fellow of the Royal College of Surgeons (FRCS). It took a lot of time and much effort to prepare for these rather intimidating examinations, and much money to afford the trip and the fees. Nevertheless, I managed to save some money from my residency salary—which most residents never get to spend because they never leave the hospital—and with a little help from my father who was still alive. My mother had died shortly after I graduated, from a bleed in the brain, and had spent three months dying in the neuro ICU.

The trip was an exhilarating experience. The weather was grey and rainy, but that didn't dampen my spirits. The Royal Colleges at Edinburgh and Glasgow go back centuries, and are the historical bastions of surgical innovations over the centuries. Just being there was an inspiring experience, and it made me acutely aware that I was to follow in the steps of so many great surgeons that walked these halls in the past.

Examinations in these colleges took about 2 months to complete; and suffice to say, I sailed through without too much incidence, and obtained the coveted title of Fellow of the Royal College, which was in effect a license to kill, much like James Bond's 007 designation. One was now legally allowed to take people into an operating room and cut them up! Quite awesome, if you think about it.

What followed was two amazing weeks, touring by train, all over Europe, before returning home to the Singapore General Hospital and being put on surgical calls the very next day.

In those days, a newly certified surgeon was immediately thrown into the deep end of the pool, so to speak. On the very first call, there was a traffic accident, and a patient came in with a ruptured spleen, which I was obliged to remove. It was an appropriate baptism of fire.

What followed was 2 years of intensive surgical practice in our busiest metropolitan hospital, which was busy daily, to overflowing, and there were merely 3 young surgeons that took turns being on call. The experience was mind boggling. It was not unusual to have to perform 10 major and 10 minor operations on every call.

Two years at this grueling pace matured a surgeon a lot, and very quickly; however, I was not satisfied to just become a normal surgeon. I wanted to contribute to the science of surgery, and I wanted to operate at the frontiers.

As such, I needed to look for the top places in the world, and train there. To do that, I had to travel once more. I was interested in therapeutic endoscopy, and researched into something new and ground breaking in surgery. I sought training in three top institutions: the Academisch Medisch Centrum, in Amsterdam; the University of Houston, in Texas; and Harvard Medical School. Of the three, I already had an offer for a fellowship at Houston, so I made plans to visit all 3 places.

The first stop was Amsterdam. The hospital was amazing, and the endoscopy service was amazing, and there were top endoscopists working there who were world famous; but no offer was forthcoming, so I made my way to the Massachusetts General Hospital, at Harvard Medical School.

I arrived on a wintery evening and called the chief of surgery at the MGH, who was the world renowned, Dr. Ronald Malt. He gave me an appointment to meet him at 5 am the next morning, at his office. I trudged through the snow and then waited outside his office, half an hour early. He came exactly on time and interviewed me for 15 minutes. He looked through my credentials and noted my already significant experience in GI endoscopy. He said, "Young man, you have excellent credentials, and I just happen to have a position in surgical endoscopy, because one fellow just indicated that he can't take up the position. The job is yours if you can get the paperwork done and be back in one month."

It was a paid surgical fellowship in surgery, with an emphasis on GI endoscopy, and also a research opportunity in basic sciences. I was appointed as Clinical and Research Fellow at the Massachusetts General Hospital and Harvard Medical School, for a 3-year stint. Dr. Malt murmured that this was the shortest interview for a job at Harvard that he had ever conducted! I returned home, and in one month, I was back working at the MGH. At this time, I was also Lecturer and Senior Registrar at the National University of Singapore, and my professor there, Prof. Foong Weng Cheong, was delighted and gave me paid leave to continue my training at Harvard. I was the first member of the Department of Surgery to have ever been sent to that amazing institution, which was then rated No. 1 in the USA, and hence, the world.

My years in Boston were some of the most enriching years of my life. It was a unique city. Everyone there was either studying something, researching something, or an expert in something. It seemed that all the intelligent people in the world were somehow congregated in this city. I basked in the environment, and absorbed everything like a sponge. My research on pancreatic cancer oncogenes didn't bear fruit. Some of the most famous names in medicine, at the time, worked at the MGH, which was nicknamed, *Man's Greatest Hospital*. When residents asked me where I came from, I would tell them SGH. They would playfully ask, "Is that the *Second Greatest Hospital?*" SGH was actually Singapore General Hospital.

My main job was to train the surgical residents, at the MGH, in gastroscopy and colonoscopy, and to perform the ERCP (endoscopic retrograde pancreatico cholangiograms), which was an endoscopic procedure where you put a scope down the throat to the duodenum, and you cannulate the bile and pancreatic ducts to inject dye into them, and visualize these ducts on x-ray. This also allowed one to remove stones from the common bile duct or stent pancreatic and bile duct tumors, to facilitate the flow of bile in blocked bile ducts. During these years, I also pursued a romance with a young lady who was studying in Toronto, Canada, which was a mere 500 miles away. We eventually got married in Honolulu, Hawaii, two years later.

I was so inspired being in Boston that I decided to pursue a 5-year PhD program in molecular genetics, which was a hot field then, because we could sequence DNA, and I was keen on using this as a platform to solving the mysteries of cancer, or developing gene therapy. I was accepted into programs in UCSF and Columbia in New York. Fortunately, my professor talked me out of it and persuaded me to remain in clinical surgery—because what was about to happen was phenomenal and shook the world.

Towards the end of my stay at Harvard, I read a small article about a new development called laparoscopic surgery. Some obscure surgeon in France was able to remove a gall bladder through tiny holes, visualizing the whole process through a laparoscope that was inserted via the umbilicus. This procedure was called laparoscopic cholecystectomy, and would totally revolutionize the entire surgical world. My boss wasn't interested at the time, and neither was anyone at Harvard. Everyone thought it was a gimmick. Prof. Malt had just invested several million dollars in a machine from Dornier, which could smash gallstones by externally applied ultrasound. A whole new center was set up to do this. Unfortunately, he bet on the wrong horse. This expensive development would not take off, but the simple technique of Dr. Phillipe Mouret, from France, would change surgery forever, and usher in the new age of laparoscopic surgery. It was time to go home and exploit this new technology.

I returned to Singapore and to clinical surgery. I had a new boss— Professor Abu Rauff. I told him about laparoscopic cholecystectomy (LC). He thought it was Mickey Mouse surgery and just a fad. He was a great and famous surgeon, of the old school, and believed in big incisions. Nevertheless, he was open minded and told me to pursue it. He was even willing to approve a small research grant to fund the equipment to do so. He didn't realize that he had just funded a surgical revolution, and that surgery in Singapore, Asia, and the world, would never be the same again.

A few months later, I was in Atlanta, Georgia, listening to Prof. Albert Cuschieri, from Dundee in the UK, give a lecture about laparoscopic surgery, and warning that this was a field only for experts who have years of experience in diagnostic laparoscopy. Next to me was a portly, red-faced German professor, who was muttering his disagreement loud enough for me to catch everything he said. In heavily German accented English, he said, "This man doesn't know what he is talking about. I can teach any surgeon to do laparoscopic cholecystectomy in 3 days!" I turned to him and told him that I would take up his challenge. He said, "Come to Cologne." In one month, I was there.

I went with my wife this time, and we passed through Paris, where I was robbed in the subway. We arrived in Cologne, penniless and without credit cards. Prof. Hans Troidl, the German pioneer of laparoscopic surgery, very generously took care of our expenses, and I spent three very productive days learning the radical technique of laparoscopic cholecystectomy.

When I got back to Singapore, the instruments and camera systems were soon delivered, and we then proceeded to do the first case, but someone in SGH had already beaten us to it. We immediately realized that this new, minimally invasive or minimal access surgery could be applied to almost every type of operation, and that the gall bladder was just the beginning.

In the same year, in Asia, we held the very first workshop on laparoscopic surgery, beating Hong Kong to it by some weeks. The next year, we started a society called the Endoscopic and Laparoscopic Surgeons of Asia, to promote this new surgery. Most of the surgeons came from regional countries, and all became pioneers in their own countries. As the first general secretary of this new organization, I wrote the constitution and registered the society, which is now one of the largest endoscopic societies in Asia, representing dozens of countries, from Turkey to Japan. The formation of this society was inspired by Dr. Gerald Marks, from the USA, who proposed that I return to Singapore and set up an Asian-wide society to promote this revolutionary type of surgery.

The development of laparoscopic surgery is described in some detail because it was the first building block in the development of surgery for diabetes. Almost all metabolic surgery today is done by a minimally invasive or keyhole technique. If we were still doing open surgery, most diabetics would probably prefer to continue with drugs or insulin. The pain and incapacity after open surgery is not to be dismissed lightly. Minimally invasive surgery greatly reduces the horror of surgery. Most times, the patients are totally comfortable the next day after surgery, and they get out of hospital the following day.

Let's get back to the story. Metabolic surgery needed another key breakthrough to reach its present state of development. It needed the development of laparoscopic stomach surgery. This needed a technique and equipment to cut and join bowel. In 1992, my team in Singapore was positioned ideally to take this step and thus get on the world stage.

From 1990 to 1992, we had done our best to find other applications for laparoscopic surgery. We successfully applied the technique to appendectomy, hernia repair, repair of perforated ulcers of the stomach and the duodenum, and vagotomy, to reduce the acid in the stomach and heal ulcers. In those days, ulcer disease still occupied much of the surgeon's time, but a paradigm shift was occurring here as well. Dr. Barry Marshall, from Perth, proved that ulcers and stomach cancer were actually due to a bacteria called Helicobacter pylori. Killing this bacteria healed most of the ulcers, and also markedly reduced the incidence of stomach cancers. In a few years, stomach surgery was about to become obsolete, except that we did not foresee that another epidemic was coming, which was going to make stomach surgery a booming field once again!

In 1991, a company based in Connecticut, USA, called US Surgical or Autosuture, invented an endoscopic stapling device that aided greatly in joining pieces of bowel together. In 1991, this device was experimental, but the developer, Peter Birtcher, decided to let me have the first 12 pieces to try. It was truly an opportunity that I couldn't pass up. I had built up a truly kick-ass team of young surgeons who were my sort of disciples, and we were truly testing the envelope. In January 1992, we started to reach for the stars. First, we removed a right colon for cancer, and reconnected the small bowel to the middle colon, totally endoscopically. Next, we removed a tumor in the left colon, and rejoined everything. Both these cases did well. The next month, we wanted to really do something that would take us into hyperspace. Till then, no one had really done a stomach resection endoscopically, with the anastomosis or reconnection done totally by endoscopy without any incision.

The previous year, Prof. Seigo Kitano had done a stomach resection laparoscopically, but he did the reconstruction through a small incision by open surgery. This was thus designated a laparoscopic assisted distal gastrectomy, or LADG. Prof. Kitano, who is one my best friends, had pioneered this. We wanted to take this to the next step. We now had the means to do a stomach resection by endoscopy, with the anastomosis or reconstruction done totally endoscopically as well, without any incision to join the gut together. This was called a totally intraabdominal gastric resection, or totally laparoscopic gastric resection.

We found a relatively thin old man with a huge bleeding gastric ulcer, and I told my team that we would do this. They thought I was mad, and everyone was skeptical. I described the methodology, and they were half convinced. I told everyone to have a good sleep that night, and the next day we just did it. It took us 3 hours for the whole operation, which was pretty fast for a world's first. Halfway through, I already realized that it was possible, and that we would complete the operation. It was being videotaped, of course; and later, I would spend more time editing this tape than doing the surgery.

When the operation was completed, and we had removed the resected stomach through a 2 cm umbilical incision, we were exhausted and stunned. We couldn't really believe what we had just achieved. It was the world's first, and it put Singapore on the surgical map of the world. That night, we had a champagne party to celebrate. The team comprised of Dr. John Isaac, Dr. Kum Cheng Kiong, and Dr. SS Ngoi, and of course, myself. The photographer was Dr. Yaman Tekant, from Istanbul.

This operation was the final stepping stone that allowed the development of all the stomach operations that are used in bariatric and metabolic surgery today. The technical advance of being able to do GI anastomosis, intraabdominally, was established on this day, the 10th of February, 1992. As they say, "The rest is history." At that time, we never even realized this. We were thinking of stomach cancer and ulcers, but we had actually laid the foundation for the development of laparoscopic bariatric and metabolic surgery.

I didn't waste time announcing our feat. I edited the video of the operation, and I submitted it to present at the upcoming SAGES (Society of American Gastrointestinal Endoscopic Surgeons) meeting, in April of 1992, in Washington DC. The program was already printed, but the organizers were so impressed by the topic of the video that they made a separate, special session in a large auditorium. The attendance at this session was beyond my wildest expectations. More than a thousand surgeons, from all over the world, crowded into the auditorium, and there were people standing both at the back and at the sides because there weren't enough seats. After showing the video, I was inundated with requests from surgeons all over the world, to visit me at the National University in Singapore. There was an overwhelming interest from surgeons all over the world, to learn this technique.

What followed were halcyon days for the next 8 years, characterized by rapid innovation, constant progress, and unbelievable excitement. Surgeons from all over the world came in a stream to the newly organized Minimally Invasive Surgical Centre (MISC), which I started in order to develop this new field of surgery in my hospital. I think it was one of the first of these types of centers worldwide. We continued to pioneer and innovate, not only in Singapore but all over the world. In 1993, I flew to Karachi, and with my friend, Mumtaz Maher, did the first thoracoscopic esophagectomy for esophageal cancer there. Only one other group, in Belgium, had reported this development at the time. We did randomized controlled trials, comparing laparoscopic and open appendectomy. We helped to pioneer mini endoscopic surgery, or needlescopic surgery, where 2 and 3 mm instruments are used to perform routine and less complex operations, with the tiniest of scars that disappear over time. We did the first thoracoscopic sympathectomies using mini instruments, and also did a randomized controlled trial, comparing mini and conventional laparoscopic cholecystectomy.

Stomach surgery, at that time, still held strong interest for me. We were extending laparoscopic gastric surgery to stomach cancer, and getting good results. Ulcer surgery was already starting to decline, and we were looking for new applications. A group of surgeons from Sicily, and another group from Brno in the Czech Republic, came to visit us because they were interested in gastric surgery for bariatric applications. Obesity was just starting to be a problem in Europe, and had not yet become a big problem in Asia. These visits and interactions clued me into the trend that bariatric surgery for obesity would be the next big thing in surgery, and that it had to be done by keyhole surgery; otherwise, the morbidity and recovery would be so daunting that few fat people would even consider surgery as an option. I also realized that we had already mastered all the techniques to do this surgery, when we developed laparoscopic gastrectomy. It was thus a small technical innovation that would open the way to the huge boom in obesity surgery.

The missing piece of the puzzle was the energy devices, which allowed the surgeon to cut through tissue, without bleeding, during endoscopic surgery. Ethicon came up with the harmonic scalpel and shears, using ultrasonic energy; Covidien, which succeeded Autosuture, came up with the LigaSure, which uses heat to seal and a cold metal blade to cut. These devices made endoscopic surgery far quicker and safer. There have been many upgrades and new devices since. During the mid-nineties, most surgeons also learnt to suture endoscopically. This is a technically demanding skill, and a surgeon can never do the more complex procedures until he can do this. The MISC ran many training courses to teach this skill at all levels, to residents and to visiting surgeons from all over the world. The equipment for suturing also became more sophisticated and more ergonomic.

At this time, I was travelling 15 to 20 times a year to attend conferences and to demonstrate advanced surgical techniques. I have done surgery in more than 25 countries in 5 continents. I missed Antarctica and Africa, but I have operated everywhere else. There were so many invitations that it was difficult to decide which ones to accept.

We also helped to propagate endoscopic surgery to the fields of lung and heart surgery, as well as spine surgery, working with our cardiac and orthopedic colleagues. It's strange how things just go round, and you end up back in the same place. Minimally invasive surgery of the spine evolved into an important field, and so did minimally invasive surgery of the chest. It got a new name: video assisted thoracoscopic surgery (VATS). It was really rewarding to help my colleagues develop these two fields in my hospital.

In the later part of the decade, we at last began to apply laparoscopic surgery to obesity. Our first patient was a middle-aged Chinese lady with a BMI of about 40. She was willing to be our first case, and we did a gastric bypass on her. This was around 1997. She did extremely well and regained her ideal weight within about 6 months. At about this time, the gastric band became popular, as it was really easy to deploy, and the surgery could be done really quickly and easily. It took the world by storm, except for the USA, which stuck to gastric bypass, much of which was being done by open surgery in the late nineties.

My final years at the MISC in the National University Hospital were somewhat turbulent, as I was involved in surgical robotics. This field never really took off because of high capital cost, and in most fields, it did not add any benefit to the patient, though it did make the task for surgeons easier in certain very specific areas like prostate surgery. I was also involved in a microrobotics project, trying to make a microrobot that could crawl up the colon and take pictures. These activities resulted in a keynote lecture at the Royal College of Surgeons in London, which was rather cool. We also did robot-assisted surgery by satellite, between Johns Hopkins Baltimore and NUH in Singapore, and one of the first robotic laparoscopic cholecystectomies in the world, and certainly the first in Asia.

In 2000, I did my finale with the National University of Singapore, by organizing the 7th World Congress of Endoscopic Surgery, under the banner of ELSA and IFSES (International Federation of Societies of

Endoscopic Surgery). I was President of the Congress, which brought more than 3000 delegates from nearly 50 countries. After this fabulous event, I resigned as Associate Professor of Surgery at the National University. The next 5 years would be in Deutschland (Germany). It was *ultra cool*, as the Germans would say.

Once again, what goes around comes around. I was once again working with Prof. Hans Troidl, the pioneer of laparoscopic surgery in Germany, and based at the University of Cologne, in Merheim. We did every kind of laparoscopic surgery, but it soon became apparent that the growth area was bariatric surgery, surgery for the reversal of obesity. We started mainly doing gastric bands but quickly transitioned to the laparoscopic Roux-en-Y gastric bypass. This operation was just gaining interest in Germany, and Prof. Stefan Saad and I did the first one together, in Cologne. The other procedure we worked on was the intragastric balloon. I inserted the first of these balloons in Cologne, and then was able to pioneer this device in Singapore, Indonesia, and Japan. While in Germany, I did some travelling for work as well, though not as prolifically as when in Singapore.

The intragastric balloon was introduced to Japan when Prof. Seigo Kitano, of Oita University, invited me to put in the first one there. It was a great honour. The Japanese, on the whole, are not obese, but they have a higher propensity to develop the co-morbidities of obesity, such as diabetes, hypertension, and heart disease, at a much lower BMI. The balloon seemed to be a good solution for this country.

During this time, bariatric surgeons all over the world began to notice that bariatric operations not only made the patient reduce weight, but that very often, their type 2 diabetes, hypertension, and high cholesterol could also disappear, along with the lost kilograms. It seemed almost magical. At first, everyone thought it was the weight loss that did the trick. We soon realized that stronger forces were at work; hence, the field of metabolic surgery was born.

Bariatric surgery was initially done for the very obese. The BMI had to be above 40. We soon noticed that if we did it for patients with a lower BMI, we reversed their co-morbidities, and this in itself was a better outcome than just losing weight. Reversing type 2 diabetes, hypertension, high cholesterol, and fatty liver was much more important than merely losing weight. Another finding was that the gastric band didn't have as much of an antidiabetic effect or metabolic effect as a bypass.

I returned to Singapore in 2005, and worked on my idea about reversing diabetes. I only had one serviceable operation to achieve this, and this was the bypass. Most people in Singapore didn't believe that their type 2 diabetes could be reversed, and there were few takers. For some years, I was a lone voice in the wilderness.

Michel Gagner came to the rescue. He developed an operation called the laparoscopic gastric sleeve resection, around 1997. It was simple and effective, and it worked for most cases. If the patient was fat, and the diabetes was not too severe, it worked beautifully. It is one of the commonest operations done in the world now. The antidiabetic effect is not as strong as a gastric bypass, but for most mild to moderate diabetics, it is a good solution.

I was invited to be part of the faculty at the Hamad Medical Corporation in Doha, Qatar, where I operated regularly for about 2 years. Michel was the head of the bariatric service, and there were 4 very talented young surgeons there, whom I helped to train. At the HMC, 95% of the operations were sleeve resection, and it was not uncommon to do 8 operations per day, running two operating rooms. With the sleeve resection, the complete remission of type 2 diabetes occurred in about 65% of the diabetic patients. The rest improved but did not reverse completely.

Back in Singapore, I continued to pursue the idea of metabolic surgery rather than just pure bariatric surgery. We did the sleeve for the mild and moderate diabetics who were obese, and chose the bypass for the more severe diabetics and the lower BMI patients. At first, we favored the Roux-en-Y; but recently, we transitioned to doing more single anastomosis gastric mini bypasses, which are simpler and seem to have the same or better results.

My efforts were rewarded by awards and recognition from Saudi Arabia, Japan, and Indonesia.

Five years ago, I decided to start globalizing, as Singapore was too small and too expensive. I felt that our techniques and technology were scalable and exportable. Having operated on some high profile people, such as several ministers, a governor from Russia, a general's wife from Azerbaijan, and a Kurdish general and warlord, I was soon able to develop bariatric and metabolic centers in these countries. Opportunities then opened up in Germany, China, and Indonesia. Recently, India opened up to us. The idea of metabolic surgery to reverse and even cure diabetes has now been embraced all over the world. A recent guideline published by the American Diabetic Association, in 2016, was endorsed by 45 medical and surgical societies worldwide. There is no longer any doubt about the effectiveness of this form of surgery.

Many of my patients were really important people. Among my patients were a prince, a prime minister, a minister of finance, several other Russian ministers, several governors and mayors, a director general of defense, an aide to a president, several generals, many members of parliament, and a large number of corporate leaders, oligarchs, and celebrities. For purposes of confidentiality, I shall not reveal their identities.

In 2011, I was appointed a Full Professor by Monash University in Melbourne, Australia, and have returned to academic life, teaching at the Clinical School in Malaysia. Concurrently, I run my private practice in Singapore and am building up all my overseas centers. I now can offer my patients surgery in 9 centers in 5 countries.

In 2017, I also started operating in Shanghai, and developed an association at The Yosemite Clinic and Yosemite Hospital. They have two hospitals, one in Pudong and one in Puxi. Bariatric and metabolic surgery is not well penetrated in China, and I was privileged to introduce its benefits to Shanghai. In July 2019, I became Chief of the Surgical Division, and also Chief of the General Practice Department in the Yosemite Group. Yosemite Group will expand to other cities in China.

Recently, I have also been asked to take my services to two centers in India, and also back to the Middle East.

I am now on the last lap of my career, and I hope to spread the gospel of metabolic surgery worldwide, and benefit as many diabetics as possible so that they may live healthy, normal lives, and enjoy a normal life expectancy. The success of this procedure should speak for itself, and I merely have to disseminate the information to you.

Please act on this information because it will give you a longer and far healthier life than if you choose to merely control your disease and live with it.

Chapter 16

Change the Game

Personal Choices

If you have diabetes today, you are fortunate.

If you lived before the 1920s and had diabetes, you invariably died. There was no treatment before Banting and Best started using insulin. From then till the late 1990s, diabetes was an incurable, lifelong disease. You either controlled it with very stringent lifestyle changes, involving strict diet and exercise regimes, or you were condemned to a life of daily medications or insulin injections. You suffered and made the pharmaceutical industry rich.

Medical treatment does not really change the statistics regarding your cardiovascular risks and cancer risks. You will still live 10 years less on the average. It is estimated that most diabetics on medical treatment are not well controlled. If you are on insulin, your life really revolves around your blood sugar levels and your insulin injections. Every small decision is clouded by this consideration.

Over the last 20 years, the game has changed. It has changed in a way that totally benefits you. Unfortunately, it didn't change in any way that benefits the doctors or the pharmaceutical industry.

Quite by chance, it had been noticed, then tested, and then verified that surgery is the magic bullet. Very simple procedures, originally designed to make patients lose weight, were astoundingly powerful tools to reverse and even cure the disease. More impressively, the diabetes reversed in days, even before any significant weight loss had occurred. As an extra bonus, all the other aspects of metabolic syndrome, like hypertension, high cholesterol, and fatty liver, all reversed with it.

This caused amazement in some circles, and dismay in others. There are always winners and losers. In this case, you, the patient, are the biggest winner of all!

The miracle didn't end there. Complications of diabetes also became arrested or reversed. The kidneys got better, the nerve problems improved or went away, and blurred vision improved overnight. This brought even more dismay to doctors treating these conditions.

Their loss is your gain. You now have the historical opportunity to reverse and cure your disease. Never has this been possible in the history of the world. Even the internet search engines are beginning to acknowledge that type 2 diabetes is no longer incurable.

It is also good to remember that the earlier you reverse your diabetes, the more successful the outcome of the operation will be. Surgery should not be regarded as the last resort treatment.

If you are on insulin, you have a very high chance of getting off injections, so your benefit is great. If you are having complications from diabetes, they may resolve or be arrested.

In 2016, the American Diabetic Association bowed to overwhelming scientific data, and finally endorsed metabolic surgery as an equal option for the treatment of diabetics, and set up guidelines. The consensus statement was very powerful and was endorsed by 45 top medical and surgical societies worldwide.

Change the Game

Metabolic surgery is now widely accepted and mainstream. Many hospitals offer it, yet patients remain ignorant and are very seldom offered this option, which is clearly the superior option.

Doctors who withhold telling patients about all the options, are actually in contravention of medical ethics in many countries. Not telling that surgery produces better results than medical treatment is also a contravention of medical ethics, because this is a scientific fact and is evidence based.

If you are a diabetic, you must be told that you have a choice. Your doctor should tell you that metabolic surgery exists. He should make it very clear that the results of surgery are better than any medical treatment, even together with lifestyle change. He should give you a choice, and your choice must be an informed choice.

This book is written for the diabetic patient. You are the most important person in this whole complicated equation. It is your life that we want to prolong. It is your disease that we should strive to cure.

Choose well, so that you may *"Live long and prosper."*

(Last quotation from *Star Trek: The Original Series*)

About the Author

Peter Goh is well known to the international medical and surgical community. Over his long, 40-year career, he has operated in more than 25 countries in 5 continents.

He was a President Scholar in Singapore, graduated at the top of his medical class, became Fellow of the Royal College of Surgeons, in both Edinburg and Glasgow, and did his higher surgical training at the Massachusetts General Hospital, Harvard Medical School, Boston.

He was Associate Professor at the National University of Singapore, Guest Professor at the University of Cologne, and Full Professor of Surgery at Monash University. He now currently holds the positon of chairman, of both the Surgical and the General Practice Department at the Yosemite Clinic and Yosemite Hospital in Shanghai. He also runs Advanced Surgical Group in Singapore, which now operates in Singapore, China, Germany, and Russia, and may soon make inroads into India and the Middle East.

Over the years, he has served as Visiting Professor in top institutions in Brazil, USA, China, Saudi Arabia, and many other countries. He has received awards from many surgical societies worldwide, and is honorary Fellow to many surgical societies. He founded the Endoscopic and Laparoscopic Surgeons of Asia, in 1991, and was founding Governor of the International Federation of the Societies of Endoscopic Surgeons.

His pioneering work in surgery includes performing the first laparoscopic Billroth II gastrectomy in the world. He also pioneered laparoscopic colon resection in Asia, performed the first laparoscopic robotic cholecystectomies in Asia, and brought mini-laparoscopic or needlescopic surgery to Brazil. He has a very long list of published peer reviewed scientific papers, and numerous book chapters in top surgical textbooks.

In 1991, he founded the Minimally Invasive Surgery Centre, at the National University Hospital in Singapore, which has trained countless surgeons from all over the world. The center remains a well-regarded, international training center for minimally invasive surgery, under the leadership of his successor, Professor Davide Lomanto.

Over the last two decades, Dr. Goh has taken over the challenge of bringing the gospel of metabolic surgery to the world, and has a mission to convince those that have metabolic disorders, such as diabetes, hypertension, and hyperlipidemia, that their condition is not necessarily incurable and lifelong. For these patients, there is the much superior option of metabolic surgery, and Dr. Goh is dedicated to bringing remission and cure, and saving millions from the severe, negative consequences of their disease.

Acknowledgements

First of all, I would like to thank Raymond Aaron for making this book possible, and Naval Kumar for mentoring the process.

Next, I would like to pay tribute to Dr. Michel Gagner for inventing the sleeve resection operation, and for including me in his team at the Hamad Medical Corporation in Doha, in Qatar. He has always been a good friend over the space of nearly three decades.

I would like to thank Dr. Robert Rutledge for inventing and promoting the gastric mini bypass operation, which is now rising rapidly in popularity and has proven to have quite amazing results.

Among my international colleagues, I would also like to commend Dr. David Cummings, an endocrinologist in Washington, USA, who strongly supports the metabolic surgery movement, despite being a non-surgeon. He is one of few.

Appreciation goes to quantum physicist, Nika Salii, for constantly encouraging me to carry on with this book, despite my very busy schedule.

My gratitude goes to Governor Sergei Voronov, and Minister Valery Neslednikov, for helping me bring metabolic surgery to Nizhny Novgorod and Moscow. My deepest thanks to Dr. Alexander Prudkov for being our partner in Yekaterinburg.

I give thanks to my old friends, Prof. Stefano Saad and Prof. Michael Korenkov, for being my close partners in Germany.

I would also like to thank Prof. Seigo Kitano of Japan, for recognizing my work in Japan, and for connecting me to all his top Japanese colleagues.

I must also mention Jorge Lenzi of Argentina, and Gustavo Carvalho of Brazil, who have been my constant inspiration and lifelong friends. Dr. Carvalho is now the worldwide spokesman for mini-laparoscopic surgery.

More recently, I am deeply grateful for the help of Dr. Keyin Song, for helping me to promote bariatric and metabolic surgery in Shanghai and all of China. He is CEO of Yosemite Clinic and Yosemite Hospital, which is poised to be at the forefront of metabolic surgery in China. A big thanks goes to Ms. Christie Zhang for putting us together.

In Shanghai, I must also thank Ms. Marie Xu for keeping my life organized.

My deep gratitude goes to Ms. Manlam Vung and Ms. Clara Lin, staff of Advanced Surgical Group in Singapore, for keeping things running during my frequent absences. This book would not be possible without their ceaseless efforts.

I would also like to express my appreciation to Ms. Marina Fursa, from Latvia, who has promoted my activities to the Russian speaking world since 2005.

I would also like to mention General Vidadi Isgandarov for promoting metabolic surgery and my work in Azerbaijan.

Deep thanks goes to Dr. Heidi Jonatan for looking after my health and connecting me with the Indonesian medical scene. She has been a constant source of amazing support.

Acknowledgements

I must also mention my corporate partner, Mr. Koh Eng Kian, for his tremendous support of Advanced Surgical Group.

I would also, at this point, like to remember all my teachers and professors, including Prof. Foong Weng Cheong, Prof. Abu Rauff, Prof. Walter Tan, Prof. Hans Troidl of Cologne University, and the late Prof. Ronald Malt of the Massachusetts General Hospital, Harvard Medical School, for their wisdom, encouragement, and support during my formative years.

Special thanks goes to my surgical team at the National University Hospital and Minimally Invasive Surgery Center, Prof. Ngoi Sig Shang, Prof. John Isaac, and Prof. Kum Cheng Kiong, for helping me to develop laparoscopic gastric surgery.

Special mention must go to Ms. Maria Tsipkin for her help with the German videos, and Ms. Maria Bun, from Canada, for her help with our corporate videos in American English.

Lastly, I would like to thank the members of my family for their encouragement and support.

My appreciation goes to my daughter, Livy Von Goh, for all the fine YouTube videos she has produced; and to my son, Gunther Von Goh, for help with my website and providing sales and marketing training for my staff.

To my son, Theodore, I would like to express my gratitude for keeping the home front well organized and calm.

Lastly, I want to mention my first wife, Ming Chew, for being the most amazing ex-wife, and for her spiritual support and material help over the years.

www.ingramcontent.com/pod-product-compliance
Lightning Source LLC
Chambersburg PA
CBHW070642220526
45466CB00001B/263